About the Author

Martica is a native Texan who is acclaimed for her innovative fitness techniques and health writing. She was awarded 1992 UK Fitness Leader of the Year by the Fitness Professionals Association and was nominated for Special Achievement in the Fitness Industry in 1994 by the Exercise Association of England. She was the 1989 British Aerobics Champion Silver Medallist.

Martica began teaching aerobics in 1983. She became certified by the American Council on Exercise (ACE) and the Aerobics & Fitness Association of America. She also holds a BA degree in Exercise Science and English Literature from America's prestigious university, Smith College.

As well as writing *CURVES* and *The 7 Minute SEX Secret*, Martica has written and self-published two highly rated instructor textbooks. She has also produced several fitness videos, including *Martica's SEXY BODY Workout* and *Perfect Curves*. Martica is also a regular fitness adviser on national TV and radio shows.

OTHER BOOKS BY THIS AUTHOR:

CURVES – The Body Transformation Strategy
(Hodder & Stoughton)

The 7 Minute SEX Secret
(Coronet)

Secrets of an Aerobics Instructor
(Artichoke & Frederick Press)

How To Be A Personal Trainer
(Artichoke & Frederick Press)

THE SQUEEZE

The Revolutionary
Mind–Body Technique
to Shape and Slim
Your Body

Martica K Heaner

Hodder & Stoughton

First Published in 1996 by Hodder and Stoughton.
A division of Hodder Headline Plc.

10 9 8 7 6 5 4 3 2 1

ISBN 0 340 666706

Photography: Colin Thomas
Mat: Fitness Pro Mat
Shoes: Avia
The Step from Forza Fitness Equipment
Weights from Weider Products
Inside Illustrations: Ian Mitchell
Design and typesetting: Sally and Behram Kapadia
Printed and bound in Great Britain by
Butler and Tanner Ltd, Frome, Somerset.

For my mom, dad, grandmother and little brother

Contents

Acknowledgements

Thank you to my wonderful agent, Darley Anderson, who has always given me support and time when I needed it. Thanks also to Bob Smith and Tara Lawrence; Rowena Webb, Dawn Bates, Rachel Bond and Melody Odusanya at Hodder & Stoughton, Heidi Henneman, Sally Wadyka, Jerry Ford and Bas Aarts and Valerie Adams at University College London (for their patience and understanding!).

Foreword

Few authors are as fluent and easy to read as Martica Heaner. In this, her latest book, she provides an invaluable guide to toning the body in a user-friendly way. Her writing style allows her to cover technical issues in a non-technical way and in a language that everyone can understand.

Strength exercises should be an integral part of all our daily programmes. They help maintain healthy bones and muscles, they keep our tendons strong and, perhaps most importantly for some people, they are an important way to burn calories. In fat-loss programmes, strength exercises improve an individual's ability to burn fat; they contribute to an increase in metabolism and create a means of improving our ability to perform daily tasks efficiently and energetically.

For these reasons this is an important book. Martica has the ability to convey these concepts in simple, effective and clear terms whilst at the same time motivating the reader to start and adhere to a regular programme.

The Squeeze contains excellent illustrations and instructions to complete a practical and easy to follow course of exercise.

Bob Smith, MA
Loughborough University
Department of Sport Sciences

Introduction

Why *The Squeeze?*

Until recently, I never realised how easy it is to get out of shape. It creeps up on you. It seems that one day you're fit and satisfied with the way you look. Then suddenly your clothes feel tight and uncomfortable. You feel a heaviness as you walk around. And you can feel an extra bit of padding on various parts of your body.

This was all a big surprise to me because I had been active all my life playing sports and taking gymnastics and dance classes. Then when I was seventeen years old I joined a local aerobics studio in Houston. Even though I felt like a klutz, I loved the adorable leotards, booming disco music and charismatic instructors. My enthusiasm was noticed and after a few months, the studio manager asked me to train to teach. So I became an aerobics instructor and personal trainer for the remainder of high school and university and throughout my twenties. For ten years I exercised for an hour or two (sometimes more) nearly every day of the week. I was in great shape.

As my career in fitness evolved, I began to spend an increasing amount of time writing articles and books on fitness, and producing fitness videos. I reached a point where I was so busy I had to cancel most of my teaching schedule.

This meant that I went from exercising two to four hours *a day* to two or three hours *a week*. I gained ten pounds, but worse, I felt flabby for the first time in my life. I suddenly experienced what all of my students over the years have experienced: the need to exercise regularly, but the lack of time to do it. After a hard day at my computer, for the first time I had to make the decision – should I exercise tonight? Before I never had the choice.

It's easy to find the motivation and the time to work out when you're paid well to do it! Now, I could opt out if something better came along – like a dinner party or a night in a soft chair curled up with my cats and a book or if I just felt too tired. Too often, I'd put it off until the next day.

Many people I'd meet would say, 'Oh you must be so fit, how much do you exercise? I was embarrassed to admit that I probably didn't even exercise as much as they did! The reality was that I was just like them, sitting on my bum working all day, with just enough energy to teach my two classes a week.

I was still very involved with fitness, only now I was talking and writing about it more than doing it. I had spent countless hours researching the latest trends for my articles, I subscribed to numerous science journals and regularly attended fitness conventions to stay at the forefront of the latest developments in fitness, I was probably more up-to-date and knowledgeable than I'd ever been. It was just that at the highest point in my fitness career, I was at an all-time physical low.

Compared to the average person, I was still in very good shape. I had, after all, been *extremely* active for about 12 or 13 years. I was still teaching. And I'd even go for the odd six-mile run. But none the less I was doing the minimal amount of exercise, and any extra was never *regular*. I was still fit. But I was also starting to get fat.

I realised I was no superhuman, I was just like everyone else. I was also heavier, flabbier and my posture had deteriorated to the point where whenever I saw pictures of myself I'd cringe because my shoulders were so slumped. I felt guilty for not exercising enough and pressure to maintain the perfect aerobic-instructor physique.

I had to get back in shape. But I couldn't go back to my old regime of teaching non-stop; I simply didn't have the hours or energy any more. I also had time against me. Before, my junk food consumption had never translated into cellulite. Now, even the slightest over-indulgence resulted in an explosion of ripples!

I knew why I was out of shape, now I just had to find the solution. My muscle mass had obviously decreased due to the natural effects of ageing and the drastic reduction in time I spent exercising. My poor muscle tone contributed to a lowered metabolism. My body was used to burning a lot more energy. If I ate anywhere near the amount of food I'd eaten for the past ten years, if it didn't get used up, it would get stored as fat. As my muscles got weaker, my body got mushier, my posture deteriorated.

I had to find an exercise programme that would compensate for all those hours when I was more cerebral than physical. But I needed something that didn't require two hours a day.

I had to figure out how to fit in the least amount of exercise *that would work* into a very busy life. That's how I developed *The Squeeze* technique.

Reshaping my Body

I knew that my problem was largely muscular, so that meant starting a resistance-training (weight-lifting) programme. Oddly enough, despite the exercise I'd done during the previous ten years of teaching, I'd never really used weights.

This is because for many years in the fitness industry, experts promoted aerobic exercise. Running, cycling, walking and aerobics were considered the best activities for weight loss and cardiovascular health. Weight training was considered less important for overall health and was left to the bodybuilders or athletes.

But now it had become widely realised that resistance training was not just for looking good. It was as important as cardiovascular fitness, crucial for preventing injuries and integral to all-round fitness. Weight lifting allowed you to control your physique in a much more time-effective way. Recent studies had shown that you could lose more fat by combining aerobic and resistance training than by doing aerobic workouts alone. And there was also new evidence showing that the more muscle tone you had, the easier it was to maintain your body shape.

So I started lifting weights.

Starting to Squeeze

I noticed an improvement in just a few weeks. My body became firmer and I felt strong. After a couple of months my posture had improved dramatically. I noticed that my more powerful muscles gave me a grace and control I'd never had before. When I ran or did aerobics now, it was less of an effort. The funny

11

thing is that I didn't increase the amount of exercise I did by much, I simply changed *how* I was exercising.

At first I simply did basic exercises with dumbbells. Then I experimented with different moves and angles and concentrated on refining the execution of each move. I focused on making each repetition as efficient as possible. I also took note of how my students performed. I realised that most people don't put their mind into their muscle. They swing their limbs, move too fast and rely on momentum rather than precise body control. They focus *out*, rather than in. For example, they view a leg lift as the leg moving the muscle, rather than the muscle moving the leg.

When I realised this, I developed a way to teach an exercise so that a student would be encouraged to concentrate on what they were doing. It was not enough for them to mimic how I performed the exercise – they needed to know precisely *how* they should position the different parts of their body during each move. They had to know when to inhale or exhale, where to focus and how to target the correct muscles. So I devised *The Squeeze*.

The Squeeze technique is a muscle-sculpting routine with weights that brings more mental focus into an exercise. It will show you how to exercise better and you'll probably see more improvements in your body than you have with other exercise routines. *The Squeeze* will lead you to the most essential parts of an exercise, showing where and how to squeeze in order to get the safest, quickest and most effective results.

Chapter 1

What You've Never Been Told

What You've Never Been Told

Everyone knows that exercise can change your body. But most people have problems seeing real, permanent results. There are two reasons for this. First, many people do the wrong type of exercise to tone up or lose weight, or they quit too soon. In my book *CURVES – The Body Transformation Strategy*, I show you how to follow and stick to the exact programme you need to follow to get fit, slim or just healthy.

The other reason people do not get what they want from exercise is because most do not truly understand all the complexities in a specific exercise. So they end up exercising incorrectly. For example, you can do a million leg lifts, but unless you know how to challenge the muscles sufficiently, you may never get your legs as toned as you'd like.

You're Only as Good as Your Teacher

In most exercise classes the music is loud, the instructor is hard to hear and time is short. In large classes a student can't get individual attention or instruction and even if they can, there are still many unqualified instructors who do not know enough about good exercise technique.

Although you can find excellent information in *technical* books and videos, these can be hard to get and difficult to read. Some popular books *seem* credible, but lack substance – they are in effect nothing more than great marketing ideas. They may have lots of pictures, but little information. This leaves you half guessing, not quite sure if you're doing the move right. Even worse, the model demonstrating the exercise may have poor form or be doing something different from the written description. Which do you follow?

A video workout is slightly easier to follow because you see the whole movement from start to finish. But you don't always get expert instruction. Celebrity-backed videos, for example, are often more hype than help.

And even though most magazines regularly feature fitness advice, it is often not thorough. Because of limited space, an entire exercise programme is often squeezed onto one or two pages. And the more pictures they use, the fewer words, the less information that can be given.

Learn Perfect Technique Now

Just because you've chosen to exercise from a book doesn't mean you have to miss out on the knowledge you need. I've constructed the exercises in this book just as I would present them if I were giving you a personal training session. Although I can't see you perform the exercise, my years of teaching have shown me how to anticipate possible mistakes. Although I can't know your individual physical strengths and weaknesses, I can show you what to do to make an exercise harder, or easier, and how to modify it if you feel strained.

The purpose of my technique is to explain everything you need to know about each exercise. I don't merely say, 'Stand with your feet apart and reach up ten times' – I explain the *position* of your ribs, *if* your arms are bent, *which* muscles are working, exactly *where* to reach, *why* you need to reach, *what it feels like* if you're reaching incorrectly, and so on.

I think you'll find this technique more fulfilling because your mind will be involved in your movement. You will learn more about the way to use your body from *The Squeeze* technique than you ever have before.

Lose Fat – Resculpt Your Body

To reshape your body, you must do two things: decrease your fat by burning calories through aerobic exercise; and increase the strength and tone of your muscles through specific body-sculpting exercises. The aerobic work can be as simple as taking a fitness class, cycling or just walking around your neighbourhood. For the rest, I will teach you the different muscle exercises you should do. In addition, at the end of the book I will give you an overall programme to follow which includes both aerobic and body-sculpting exercises. This programme is very time effective. You only need to do *The Squeeze* exercises for 20–40 minutes two or three times a week.

The muscle-sculpting exercises I give you use weights. Don't worry if you've never even picked up a weight before. They are very easy to use and won't turn you into Arnold Schwarzenegger! You may start doing the exercises *without* weights at first to master *The Squeeze* technique. But weights are the secret tool for a firmer, better body in less time, so it's a good idea to invest in some.

The Squeeze will not only allow you to spend less time exercising, but also you will – in just a few weeks – see improvements in posture, muscle tone, body shape and overall stamina. Your legs will become toned, not jiggly. Your buttocks will lift, not sag. Your abdomen will become firm, not flabby.

The Squeeze technique is safe for all fitness levels and ages. If you have any physical injuries or weakness, however, please get your doctor's approval to follow these exercises.

You don't have to join a gym to use fancy equipment, you can do all these exercises in the privacy of your home. Even if you do decide to work out in a health club, you will feel much more confident because you will have learned how to exercise properly.

The Squeeze is based on sound physiological and kinesiological principles, and incorporates the latest scientific research on the mind–body connection. Most importantly, it *works*.

Chapter 2

The Mind–Body Connection

The Mind–Body Connection

The relationship between the body and mind is very powerful. In one sense, it's obvious. Your brain is the command centre of every physical function. Every movement of the body originates in the brain. But it goes deeper than that.

Research into the links between the brain and body is finding that the way you think and feel affects your body too. You can see this in immediate bodily reactions to fears and thoughts. You're scared, so your heart beats faster. You're nervous, your palms get sweaty. You're sad, you cry. You're depressed, you become listless and tired.

The physical effects of negative thoughts and emotions are even greater. More and more research is showing how mental stress can wreak havoc on the body. If you are anxious or depressed, your immune system is weakened, making you susceptible to disease and illness. It seems that a sick mind can create a sick body.

And the converse is true as well. If your body is not well, your mind can be affected. If you are nutritionally deficient, you can become depressed, tired, apathetic, or impatient. If your body is physically weak or if you have chronic pain, it can affect you mentally. The mind and body are so integrally related that determining which affects the other is a bit like the chicken and the egg. What is not in doubt is that the body and mind can affect each other positively as well.

A Healthy Body Means a Healthy Mind

It's clear that exercise makes a healthier body. What is only now being realised, however, is that exercise can also make a healthier mind. One neuropsychologist found that after four weeks of aerobic exercise, rats averaged a 20 percent increase in the number of blood vessels nourishing the brain. At the very least this means a greater oxygen supply. Clearly there are distinct physiological changes which can affect mental abilities and psychological well-being.

Studies have also shown improved mental abilities in those who exercise. Many corporations are now investing in fitness programmes for their employees because fit workers tend to work harder, longer and more effectively. One study showed that after participating in a regular exercise programme, workers committed 27 percent fewer errors on tasks involving concentration and short-term memory. NASA found that compared to the average office worker, whose efficiency decreases 50 percent for the final two hours of the working day, exercise adherents worked at full efficiency all day, amounting to a 12.5 percent increase in productivity. At the very least, improved health means that an employee who feels better will probably work better. Physical activities which require coordination skills also seem to keep that part of the brain active, a part which naturally deteriorates with ageing.

Research has also shown that *any* exercise can improve mood. Most exercisers report that they feel better during and after a workout session. It has been proved that often there are *immediate* decreases in anxiety. And over the long term, exercise has also been shown to help alleviate depression and improve self-esteem.

How does this happen? Exercise is simply controlled stress on the body. The body reacts to this stress by adapting, becoming stronger. For this to take place, a host of physical changes take place within the muscles and throughout the whole body, including the brain. Clearly a stronger body can handle more physical stress. But it appears that a certain mental toughening up results from exercise as well. This can be explained by:

Feel-Good Hormones: Exercise helps regulate hormone release in the body. Most people have heard of the hyped up 'aerobic high'. This is a euphoric state which is brought on by the release of beta-endorphins, a morphine-like hormone, in the blood and brain. Although most studies show that you can only experience the true aerobic high (where you feel as if you're floating on air) after 60–90 minutes of intense exercise, even moderate workouts can produce feel-good tingles. Consider the pleasurable release of tension you feel when you stretch in the morning or the waves of highly-charged energy you get during a motivating aerobics workout or bike ride.

But pleasure hormones aren't the only side-effects of exercise. When you exercise, your heart rate, blood flow and overall metabolism speed up. Research indicates that exercise uses up excess stress hormones like cortisol and it is this lack of 'bad' hormones which helps you feel better.

Increased Alpha Waves: Exercise is also associated with increased alpha waves in the brain. These waves are electrical patterns of brain activity which indicate that the mind is relaxed. Normally the brain is in this state upon awakening and just before sleep. This pleasurable state of consciousness is associated with positive emotions like peace, hope and happiness. Meditation and exercises with a mindful element like yoga or tai chi are also said to alter brain-wave patterns favourably. What surprises many people is that a hard run or a strenuous workout with weights can have the same effect.

Improved Body Systems: Regular exercise stimulates the nervous system and the activity of various neurotransmitters which are associated with mood changes. Neurotransmitters are chemicals which transmit impulses from a nerve cell to another cell to start or stop an action.

But the mental changes induced by exercise can't always be detected by physiological measures. At the very least, physical effort can provide a sort of physical release for mental stress and excess tension. Although a hard workout can be exhausting, an experienced exerciser will swear by its exhilarating effects. Or it could be that exercise is a placebo and the mental benefits are due to psychological reasons. For example, physical activity and regular training allow you to set and attain small short-term goals. This provides a sense of achievement which can give you a sense of control over your life which in turn may help improve self-confidence. Improvements in body shape and physical skills can also lead to improved self-esteem.

The Mind–Body Connection

Whatever the scientific explanation, the simple fact is that exercise makes you feel better both physically and mentally.

Thinking with Your Muscles

Because so much is still unknown, there are ongoing debates about which type, how much and how intense the exercise must be to affect mood. In fact, all types of exercise, from high intensity aerobics to slower muscle conditioning and stretching, appear to produce psychological benefits. Certain types of exercise seem more disposed to providing mental benefits. These include yoga, swimming, running, walking and tai chi. The key ingredient seems to be that these exercises have a mindful component or meditative effect. By adding a mindful component you attain an internal awareness which stimulates the mind–body connection. Where your attention goes, your energy follows. This has a revitalising effect.

Which Activities Make You Feel Good?

You can adopt a mindful approach to *any* exercise. If you focus in, rather than focus out, no matter what you are doing, you will develop an inner awareness that can enhance the way you feel. Like a puppy running full speed in a field or a cat luxuriating in a morning stretch, you'll recognise how good it feels simply to move your body. Training the mind as well as the body can be as simple as pure meditation practised during yoga, deep breathing during a stretch class or focused concentration during a weight-lifting workout. Certain repetitive exercises like running and swimming can produce this calming effect as well. It's the mental aspect which has been shown to produce the psychological benefits.

Many athletes strive for an altered state of consciousness known as a *peak flow* mental state. After hours of refining every aspect of their skill and visualising every part of their performance, they reach a state of hyperfocus. Their movement becomes effortless. Suddenly they are so 'in the moment' that they experience timelessness – ten seconds can seem like ten minutes. They become unaware of any distractions. This can happen in a tennis match or a triathlon. It can happen in a race, a round of golf or a football match. Players who have described reaching this moment have said that it occurs in winning performances, when they are playing up to or surpassing their potential. Their ability to focus enables them to attain excellence.

- *The Squeeze* technique is a more mindful approach to body exercises. Instead of swinging your arms and legs frantically in different directions, you will control your movement with mental focus. And as well as seeing a firmer, stronger body, you will find that the exercises have a calming effect on the mind.

- But you don't have to be a professional athlete to experience this mind–body connection. All you need to do is do your regular exercises in a more thinking way.

Chapter 3

Train Your Brain

Train Your Brain

Focusing your mind in your workouts can not only help you feel good, it can also improve your results.

Try making a fist. Now bend your arm back and forth at the elbow, first quickly, then slowly. This is a biceps curl. Now pretend you are holding a 25 lb (11 kg) weight in your hand and consciously tighten the muscle in the front of your upper arm. Bend and straighten your arm again. You will notice a tremendous difference between the two. When you focused on the movement, suddenly the muscle felt more resisted, didn't it? There was no actual increase in weight, but you worked the muscle harder and had more control over the action. By feeling your arm, your muscle and its movement through space, you were able to focus and *squeeze* at the core of the action. This gave you a control that just swinging your arm back and forth never could.

Notice that part of the exercise involved your imagination. You *imagined* that you were holding a weight. There is a fascinating reason why this helped you. Research into the working of the mind has shown that the brain does not have the ability to distinguish between real and imagined actions. If you picture yourself holding a weight when you are not, then some of the body changes which occur when you do it in reality actually take place. In other words, your brain sends the same messages to your muscles. More muscle fibres are recruited and fired up. You could feel the difference in mus-

cle force generated between biceps curl one and biceps curl two. No physical change caused this, just the mental intervention.

One study recently asked a group of people to do leg extension exercises to strengthen the front of their thighs. Another group was asked not to move at all, simply to imagine themselves doing the exercise. Not surprisingly the group doing the exercises showed an increase in muscle strength. Amazingly, so did the group who visualised. Of course this doesn't mean you can just lie back and think yourself thin! But thinking about what you're doing clearly can enhance the effectiveness of your workout.

Another study found that subjects performed 145 percent more push-ups and pull-ups in half the time when they did them themselves as opposed to when they were coached. When on their own, they sped up and were able to do more than when they were led through the exercises at the exact same speed. When they were listening to their body and controlling it, they were better able to meet the challenge than when their focus was directed outwards. Many other studies have also shown that mental preparation which enhances personal focus can have profound effects on performance.

This personal focus is the basis of *The Squeeze* technique. Rather than go on automatic pilot, you'll focus on your body and involve your mind. This will allow you to maintain proper form and increase the tension of the muscles to make them work harder without straining yourself.

Mind Skills

Your mind–body skills are already more advanced than you think. We all have a natural instinct to determine how we feel and to control the body.

In the 1960s Swedish exercise physiologist Dr Gunnar Borg discovered that we have a highly accurate barometer for determining how we feel. He tested people of different fitness levels working out at different intensities. At various points he would ask them how hard they felt they were working. Their answers could range from feeling their workout was 'very light' to 'somewhat hard' or 'very heavy'. At the same time as they described their feeling, he measured their heart rate. From it he determined at what percentage of their maximum capacity they were working.

Oddly enough, Borg found a direct correlation between the subjects' real and perceived levels of exertion. If they felt they were working 'somewhat hard', he found that they were all consistently working at the same level of difficulty or at the same percentage of their maximum heart rate. In other words, although the subjects were all of different fitness levels, they could accurately perceive their own appropriate level of exertion. From this Dr Borg devised a scale that is still widely used in most exercise classes and fitness-testing situations. His research made clear just how accurate the human barometer is and how much instinctive knowledge an individual has about their body.

Visualisation

The act of mentally picturing or verbalising something you wish to happen can help it happen. This is not only the principle behind positive thinking in order to lead a happier life, but is also the basis of natural self-healing techniques where, for example, a patient imagines his cancer tumour shrivelling up. By visualising an event, the brain kick starts into action some of the body processes involved.

The key to visualisation is to be as specific as possible. Not only do you think about the event, you think about it in every detail. If you are imagining yourself performing in a race, imagine how each step of the race will feel, how parts of your body will feel, the sensations of the crowd around, the noises you hear, what you see or smell. Try to reproduce the positive emotions and sensations associated with the activity and see yourself getting stronger, looking better. Produce as much feeling in the image as possible. You can apply this technique to anything really. Just remember to keep the picture vivid.

In *The Squeeze* technique I want you to apply visualisation and focusing techniques to your exercises. When you're exercising, be conscious of how your body moves and how the space around you, the ground you're on and your muscles contracting feel. I will give you key body parts to focus on during each exercise. This will help you get a sense of the whole body and how it interacts with the individual muscle group you are working.

In the next few chapters you'll learn more about how your muscles work. This will enable you to exercise with a greater understanding of what is happening.

Chapter 4

Your Body, Your Muscles

Your Body, Your Muscles

Truly understanding your muscles – and how they work – is the key to *The Squeeze*. What enables us to perform any type of movement at all is our muscles. Without them we would collapse in one big skeletal heap. Without their finely coordinated movements we would walk like robots. Some of us would be skin and bone, others pure flab.

Muscles are the support system of the body. They connect our bones together so we can move. The junction of two or more bones is known as a *joint*. A muscle attaches to different points around a joint. A strong muscle can support weight and absorb much of the force that a joint may be subjected to. Strong, well-balanced muscles protect the weaker structures within a joint.

For example, one of the biggest muscle groups in the body is the quadriceps (see illustration, page 33). This is a group of four muscles on the front thigh which join together to form attachments on each end. The lower end is attached to the upper part of the shin bone, below and to the outside of the knee. It also attaches just above the knee. The upper end is attached to the pelvis above the thigh bone. When part of the muscle contracts or shortens, it causes the entire lower leg to straighten at the knee. You can feel your quadriceps tighten if you straighten your leg. When this muscle group is relaxed, the fibres lengthen so

you can bend your knee. It's almost as if our bodies are like marionettes and our muscles are the strings.

When your quadriceps are strong, they provide excellent protection for the fragile knee joint. They help hold your kneecap in place. If you were to be kicked, or fall and twist this area, a strong muscle could give you stability to resist the strain, or at least minimise the intensity of the injury. Strong quadriceps also give the thigh its shape and keep it feeling firm and looking toned.

Muscles generally work in opposing pairs: when one shortens, the other lengthens. With *The Squeeze* technique it is important to work all the muscles in your body, not just a targeted few, to achieve muscular balance.

Moving Your Muscles

Muscles come in different shapes and sizes and they move in different directions. Big muscles tend to execute powerful, large movements. Think of the thighs and buttocks which allow you to jump and run. Small muscles execute refined, precise movements. Think of the muscles in the foot and hand or around the neck. The joints where we can perform an elaborate range of movement, such as our shoulders and hands, tend to have many different muscles to coordinate complex actions.

For example, the shoulder blades are two bones in the upper back which are involved in most arm movements. More than eight different muscles initiate the actions which move the shoulder blades up and down, forwards and backwards, towards or away from the spine, or slightly rotated in different directions. You can imagine that if one of these muscles is weak, the shoulder blades could be slightly off-kilter. This might not only affect your ability to perform certain movements, but could also lead to postural injuries. If you have slumped shoulders, it may simply be due to weak rhomboids, the muscles in between the shoulder blades (see illustration, page 30).

You can tell in which direction a muscle will contract by looking at where it is attached and the line of the muscle fibres. Most anatomical drawings will lightly sketch these in. So if a muscle attached to your spine has fibres that run horizontal to your body, then you know this muscle will rotate the spine.

While it's not *vital* to know this, it can help you determine how effective an exercise is. For example, many years ago, a very popular exercise for the waist was to stand up and twist your ribcage right and left as fast and as hard as you could. No doubt some people still do this, thinking that they are whittling away inches around their middle. If you look at pages 34–35 to see the muscles around the waist, however, you'll see that the main muscles there have fibres that run mostly vertically and diagonally, not horizontally. The muscles cause you to bend forwards (as in a sit-up) or across (as when you bring your shoulder to your opposite knee), *not* in a horizontal twisting motion. In fact, the twisting action is not caused by these muscles in the waist area at all, but by deep muscles near the spine. So when you do this twisting exercise, you are working your back and can overstress your spine. Your waist is hardly affected at all.

By knowing the shape and position of muscles' fibres, you can also tell what a muscle *can't* do. For example, many people think that doing side leg lifts will tone the outside of the upper thigh. In fact there is no muscle here (see illustrations, pages 32–34). Your buttocks actually initiate this movement. Any excess flesh on your outer thighs is fat, not muscle.

Some muscles have fibres that run in several directions. This means that a portion of the muscle may be used during certain actions. When you train these muscles, it's a good idea to vary the exercises you do and the angles you work at, so you target as much of the muscle as possible. I have accounted for this in the exercises I have selected for you.

How a Muscle Contracts

Knowing how your muscles contract will help you perform your exercises with greater control.

As a muscle shortens it exerts force. Your brain determines how hard a muscle must work. Sometimes this is based on prior experience. You look at a watermelon, for example, and know it is heavy. Even though a pillow may *look* bigger, you know it is lighter. The brain sends its signals through nerves attached to a muscle. A nerve and all its attached muscle fibres is called a *motor unit*. One motor unit can comprise two or three, a couple of hundred or even several thousand muscle fibres. To lift the watermelon, your brain will activate more motor units than it will to lift a pillow.

When the brain sends a signal to the nerve, all the muscle fibres attached to that nerve will contract 100 percent. But most muscles have many nerves and therefore many different motor units. Not all motor units in a muscle are activated for every movement. The amount of force needed to perform a particular action will determine how many motor units are used.

When you exercise a muscle, it exerts the

appropriate amount of force needed for a particular action. When you write with a pencil, the muscles in your arms exert enough force to hold it so you won't crush the lead. This is a great deal less than what would be required to hold a bowling ball. If you are moving furniture, your muscles will recruit more units in an attempt to exert a strong enough contraction to provide the necessary force. But if the object is too heavy, you might not be strong enough to move it.

The most effective way to train a muscle is to try to work as many motor units as possible. This might mean doing an exercise in different positions or using greater amounts of resistance. After a period of regular training, you'll become stronger and will fatigue more slowly so you last longer. This is because your muscle learns to recruit more motor units, the coordination of several motor units firing at once improves and there is an increase in how frequently the motor units contract. The more conditioned you are, the more quickly you will be able to recover from one contraction and do another. These, and other neurological changes, are responsible for your improved muscle strength, efficiency and control when you exercise.

Getting in Touch with Your Muscles

Look at each of the following illustrations and compare it to your own body. Trace the outline of the muscle on your body so you get an idea of its size and shape. Then read the description and contract the muscle so you can feel it working.

There's no need to memorise the muscle names, this is just an exercise so you can become familiar with parts of your body. Knowing exactly how your muscles move will help you perfect your exercise technique. By learning the action each muscle performs, you can look at any exercise and determine which

muscles are working. In general, there are opposing muscle groups on either sides of a limb. When one side contracts, the other will relax, and vice versa.

A muscle will shorten to move the bones it is attached to in a particular direction. This is known as the *concentric* contraction. The same muscle will then remain slightly contracted as the bones move back to their original position. This is known as the *eccentric* phase of the contraction. I will discuss these two different types of contraction later in the book. For now, just be aware that the muscle acts in this way.

In each exercise, I have left out some of the smaller, deeper muscles because they are difficult to feel. You may notice them on the illustration. Just note that many muscles work together to perform an action. Some of them cause the bones to move, while others hold surrounding bones in place to help stabilise the body.

UPPER BODY

Arms

Triceps

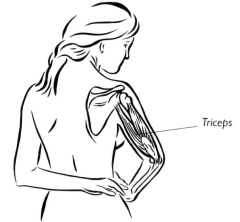

Triceps

Fig. I

This muscle is in the back of your upper arms.

Place your hand on the back of your arm, then bend and straighten your arm. This muscle tightens or hardens (contracts) when you straighten your arm.

Biceps and Brachialis

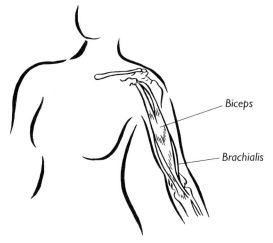

Biceps

Brachialis

Fig. 2

These muscles are in the front of your upper arms.

Place your hand on the front of your arm and bend and straighten your arm. Hold it flexed 'Popeye-style' and turn your wrist in different directions to feel how different parts of the muscle are activated at different joint angles. These muscles contract when you bring your hand to your shoulder.

Wrist Flexors/Extensors

There are several muscles in the front and back of your forearm which are involved in wrist action.

Grasp the middle of your forearm and move your wrist back and forth. Notice the muscles on top tightening as your hand bends

back, then notice the muscles underneath the forearm contracting as your hand drops forward.

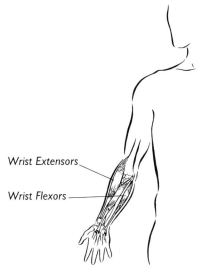

Wrist Extensors

Wrist Flexors

Fig. 3

Deltoid

This muscle group is directly on top of your shoulder. When it's well developed it gives you a nice rounded shape like a shoulder pad.

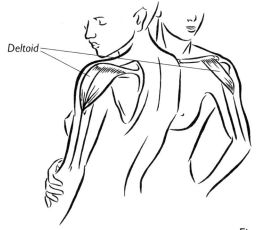

Deltoid

Fig. 4

Your Body, Your Muscles

Cup your hand on the edge of your shoulder then lift your arm directly up in front of you, out to the side and then behind you. You can feel different parts of the muscle initiating the movement in each direction. This muscle raises your arm in different directions when it contracts.

Back

Trapezius

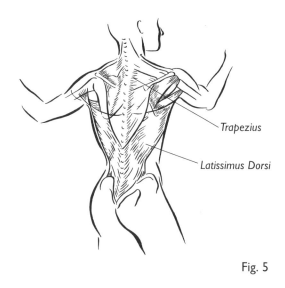

Fig. 5

This muscle is a triangular-shaped one covering most of your upper back. Because it covers such a wide area, you can feel it in several different places.

Place your hand on your shoulder in between your neck and the rounded part of your shoulder. Lift your arm up to the side. Then place your hand on your back underneath your armpits, reach your hand out to the side and pull it back in. Finally, place your hand on the lower part of your ribcage on your back and reach up. This muscle contracts whenever you lift your arm up and bring it back towards your body. It holds your shoulder blades in place.

Rhomboids

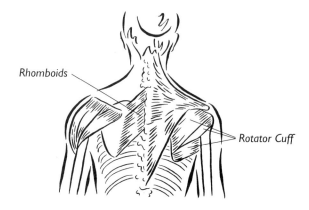

Fig. 6

These muscles are between your shoulder blades.

Reach behind your back and place the back of your hand in between your shoulder blades on your upper spine. Now lift your elbows out to the sides, keeping them shoulder level, then pull your arms back behind you. These muscles contract and move the shoulder blades towards and away from each other.

Latissimus Dorsi (see fig. 5)

This muscle covers a very large area of your back.

Reach underneath your arm and place your hand flat on top of the back ribs. Reach your hand out in front of you and pull the elbow back in to your ribs. This muscle contracts whenever you stretch out and pull in towards the body.

Rotator Cuff (see fig. 6 and 7)

This small group of muscles lies in and around the shoulder joint.

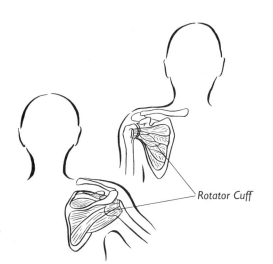

Fig. 7

Erector Spinae (see fig. 8)

These muscles run along both sides of your spine from top to bottom.

Place your hand on the middle or lower spine and slowly bend forward, then straighten back up to an erect position. These muscles contract when your spine bends and straightens. They also play a large role in stabilising your back for perfect posture.

Chest

Pectorals

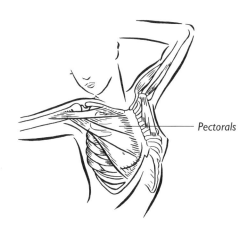

Fig. 9

These muscles are connected to your upper arm and breastbone. Place your hand on the junction on the front side of your underarm where your shoulder and torso meet. Move your arm across your chest towards the opposite shoulder.

Quadratus Lumborum

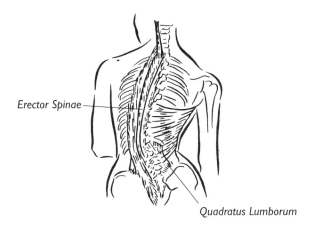

Fig. 8

This muscle is in the lower back, but is deep and so difficult to feel.

Place your fingers along the outer edge of your spine in the lower back. While your back is straight, press your fingertips deep into the muscle. Then bend to the side and back up to feel this muscle contract.

Your Body, Your Muscles

LOWER BODY

Calves

Gastrocnemius

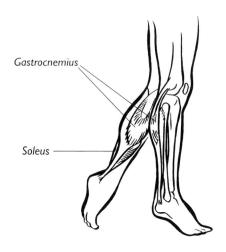

Fig. 10

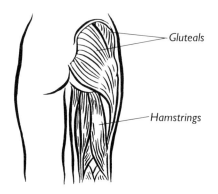

Fig. 11

This muscle is in your calf.

While standing, reach down and place your hand on the back of your lower leg. Lift your body weight on your toes so that your heel rises to feel this muscle contract. It is the rounded muscle at the top of your calf.

Soleus (see fig. 10)

This muscle is in the front of your gastrocnemius.

In the same position as above, place your hand lower on your calf, just above your ankle. Lift your heel up and down to feel the muscle contract.

Thighs

Hamstrings (see fig. 11 and 12)

This is a group of three muscles in the back of your thighs: the biceps femoris, the semitendinosus and the semimembranosus.

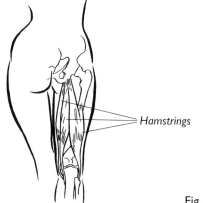

Fig. 12

Stand up and place your hand on the back of your upper leg, then bend your knee. Lift your heel to your buttocks to feel these muscles contract.

Quadriceps (see fig. 13 and 14)

This group in the front of your thigh is one of the biggest in the body and consists of four muscles: the rectus femoris, the vastus medialis, lateralis and intermedius.

Place your hand on the front of your thigh.

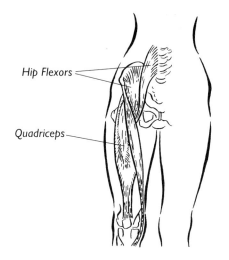

Hip Flexors

Quadriceps

Fig. 13

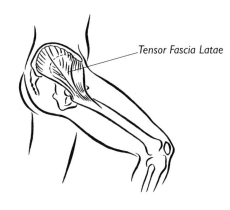

Tensor Fascia Latae

Fig. 15

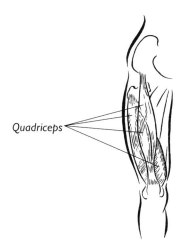

Quadriceps

Fig. 14

Bend and straighten your knee, then lift and lower your thigh to feel these muscles contract.

Tensor Fascia Latae

This muscle runs from the hip to the thigh.

Lie on your back. Place your hand on the outer hip between the hip bone and upper thigh. Then lift your leg while turning it in to feel the muscle contract.

Adductor Group

These are five muscles in the inner thigh: the pectineus, the gracilis, the adductor brevis, longus and magnus.

Place your hand on the inside of your upper leg. Then lift your thigh and move it across to your opposite hip to feel these muscles contract.

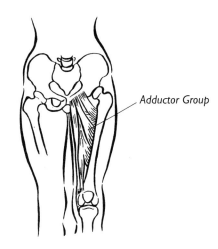

Adductor Group

Fig. 16

Your Body, Your Muscles

Hip Flexors (see fig. 13)

These muscles are in the front of your thigh, joining your upper leg and pelvis. They include the iliopsoas and sartorius.

Place your thumb on the crease between your upper thigh and pelvis. Lift your knee and thigh up towards your chest. You will notice two separate muscles. The one on the outside is the sartorius, the other is the top of your quadriceps (thigh muscles). The iliopsoas are deeper within the pelvis.

Buttocks

Gluteus Medius, Minimus, Maximus

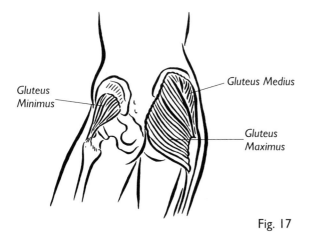

Fig. 17

These muscles give our buttocks their nice rounded shape.

Stand up and place your hands on your bum and tilt your pelvis forward and back. Then lift your leg to the side, then to the back. Finally, bend your knees as if you were about to sit in a chair, lower your hips to knee level, then straighten back up. You can feel your muscles working during all these actions.

TORSO

Abdominals

Rectus Abdominus

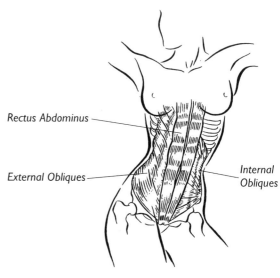

Fig. 18

This muscle is the rippled-looking one that runs along the front of your torso from your ribs to your pubic bone.

Lie on your back and place one hand just above and the other hand just below your belly button. Now lift your shoulder off the ground to feel the muscle contract. Notice how the contraction is stronger in the upper part. Next bring your knees to your chest and tilt your pelvis forward. Notice that again, the whole muscle is contracting, but the lower end is working more.

Transversus Abdominus (see fig. 19)

This muscle is the deepest abdominal muscle.

Place your hand flat on your lower abdomen. Make a cough or quick exhaling sound to feel this muscle pull the abdominal contents in.

Internal & External Obliques (see fig. 18 and 19)

These muscles run diagonally in both directions from your hips to the opposite ribs.

Lie on your back and place one hand on the right side of your lower ribcage. Place the other hand just above the left hip bone and press in slightly. Now bring your right shoulder towards your left hip to feel the muscles contract.

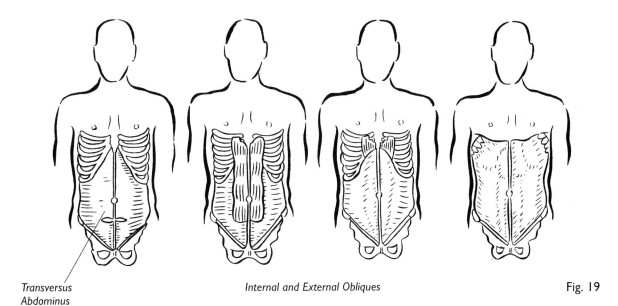

Transversus Abdominus

Internal and External Obliques

Fig. 19

Chapter 5

Sculpting Your Body

Sculpting Your Body

Every muscle has its own unique shape. You can enhance the curves of your body by training all your muscles. To sculpt your body you need to make the muscles stronger and firmer, but you also need to decrease the body fat around each muscle so that you can see its contour and definition. To achieve this you need to train your body in two different ways. I'll call the two types of movement *whole body* and *individual* exercise.

Whole body exercise incorporates activities which use many muscles, your whole body at once. These include aerobic exercises such as running, cycling, swimming, aerobic dance, stepping, skating and others. But sports like tennis, badminton, rugby, football, netball and dance are also considered whole body. Whole body exercise means you are using your body in a very functional way. You run, skip, jump, reach and throw. You perform natural actions.

By training this way, your whole body becomes fitter. But the fitness you develop is muscular and cardiovascular *endurance*, achieved not by focusing on one specific muscle, but by being active overall. Some whole body activities favour certain muscle groups – swimming uses more of the upper body, while running and cycling use more of the lower body, for example – but they still use groups of muscles to move. You do need a certain degree of strength and stamina in individual muscles to be able to do whole body exercises easily, but the focus is on the whole, not the specific.

Whole body exercise can help muscles to become stronger and firmer, but the real focus is on overall endurance. So you can't train a specific muscle for strength. One major benefit is that because you are exerting a lot of energy to carry your body around, whole body exercise tends to burn many calories so is helpful for losing weight.

Individual exercise refers to specific moves you do to train certain parts of the body. Individual exercises are sit-ups or press-ups or leg lifts in which you isolate one or a few muscles and work them very intensely to help them become stronger. Doing these exercises will not burn as many calories as running for the same amount of time, but they will help you to reshape your body, improve your posture and develop strength and muscle tone.

TYPES OF EXERCISE

Whole Body	Individual
running	abdominal crunches
tennis	push-ups
step aerobics	biceps curls
ballet	plié
walking	squats

For a well-balanced programme you need to do both types of exercises. In my book *CURVES*, I show you how to develop an overall programme of both whole body and individual exercises. In *The Squeeze*, I give you individual exercises which target all the key muscles in your body. In Chapter 12 I also give you a programme of whole body exercises to include with this routine. Both books will give you a thorough understanding of how your body works and the best way to work it.

Strength and Endurance

Strength is the amount of force a muscle can produce. If you're strong, you can lift heavy weights. *Endurance* is a muscle's ability to contract repeatedly over a period of time. This means you have the stamina to keep an activity up for a long period of time before getting tired.

It's important to recognise the difference between the two because traditionally most fitness exercises have concentrated on developing endurance, not strength. Since strength changes cause a muscle to become more firm and sculpted than endurance changes, if you haven't experienced the desired toning effects you've wanted from exercise, it may simply be that you've been developing endurance, not strength. If you're trying to develop tone, doing leg lift after leg lift after leg lift is probably a waste of time. The ability to do an exercise repeatedly does not mean your muscle will look more sculpted. In fact, it's usually the opposite because endurance work develops the slow twitch fibres which make up the muscle and neglects the fast twitch fibres which are more likely to affect muscle shape.

Strength is much more important than endurance for protecting your joints. For example, abdominal exercises are known to be good for helping to support the lower back. Some people can do hundreds of half sit-ups (also known as crunches), no problem. But more is not necessarily better. Stamina doesn't mean strength. A recent study measured subjects who could perform hundreds of repetitions of abdominal exercises. Although the high number of repetitions showed they had good abdominal *endurance*, many of the subjects had very little abdominal *strength*.

Strength and endurance are two separate aspects of muscle fitness. You must train in two different ways to develop both. Strength is developed by doing individual exercises like those in *The Squeeze*. The only way to get stronger is to use resistance on your muscles. Weights are the easiest form. Endurance is developed by doing whole body exercise, or individual exercise at a very low intensity (without using weights, for example).

Shaping Your Body

When you train for strength, you often can change the size, look and feel of a muscle. The stronger you are, the more *toned* the muscle fibres become. This means you'll feel firmer and jiggle less!

You can also change the look of a muscle by increasing its *definition*. In other words, you can make the muscle shape more visible if you decrease your body fat at the same time as improving the tone.

You can increase the *size* of a muscle, too, but this is nothing to be scared of. Slightly bigger muscle fibres are responsible for creating sinewy curves on your body. How big you can become and the shape of your muscles is largely genetic. But if you are afraid of transforming into Mr Universe, remember that no matter how hard you work, only half of 1 percent of the *male* population has the potential to develop those vein-popping bulges. Since women tend to have even less muscle mass (especially in the upper body) and less testosterone, it's extremely difficult to look like a bodybuilder. You'd have to try very hard – hours and hours of training each week using seriously heavy weights and often taking steroids or other muscle-building substances. So don't worry.

The Overload Principle

Many people do not realise that you can train your muscles in several different ways. That's why one type of training or one exercise does not develop all-round fitness. Just because you have strong arms doesn't mean they have the stamina to swim long distances. On the other hand, a runner may have incredible endurance in his legs, but this does not mean that he is strong or able to jump powerfully. It's important to do exercises for both strength and endurance.

However you train, to see progress you must use *the overload principle*. This means you must put gradual, progressive stress on your body. For example, you might start out walking for ten minutes. When this becomes easy, you overload a bit – walk faster for ten minutes or keep up the same pace but walk a little longer.

The principle is the same for individual exercises. You may start off doing five abdominal crunches. When these become easy you may do two or three more. Your body will become stronger to adapt to the new challenge. As your muscle gets stronger you overload with a few more. But remember, there is a fine line between strength and stamina. If you want to become firmer, you need to train for strength. You need to challenge the muscle to exert *more* force, not to exert the same amount of force for a longer period.

When you first do any exercise you may experience slight gains in strength. But if the exercise does not become progressively more challenging, there will be no further increase.

So you may need to do more and more repetitions to feel fatigued. This means you end up increasing only your endurance. In fact, you'll see faster, better results by lifting heavier weights for a shorter period of time.

Although if you do very many repetitions you may feel a burning sensation and think that you are working your muscles very hard, what you feel is simply a build-up of waste products in an area, not true fatigue from working the muscle to exertion. When you hold a body part in a set position and repeat a particular movement over an extended period of time, you occlude some of the blood flow to the area. As the muscle contracts it produces wastes like lactic acid which are not carried away. It's nothing serious – the minute you stop the exercise, blood flow goes back to normal and the pain subsides. But this type of stimulation is not enough to elicit the physiological changes needed to bring about improvements in strength.

Research shows that to get stronger, a muscle must be stimulated intensely for 30–90 seconds. This is the length of time is takes to complete about 8–15 repetitions, or one set of an exercise. The muscle should be challenged to the point of fatigue by the last repetition.

What does this feel like? You should feel as if it would be very difficult to perform another repetition. You may not feel any burning sensation, only weakness in the muscles. You may feel them quivering and find it difficult to perform another exercise. It can feel like your arm suddenly gives out.

But if the stimulus is too light, if you are not exerting too much effort, then you may feel perfectly fine after 15 reps. You may be able to do 10, 20, or 30 more before you feel tired. This is where most people go wrong, relying on working at a very low intensity and repeating the exercise over and over. You won't experience the best gains in strength and sculpting this way.

Getting the Balance Right

Many people concentrate on a few key muscles and ignore all the rest. Women might exercise the abdomen and buttocks to death, but neglect their back and upper body. Some bodybuilders focus on developing huge muscles in their arms and chest, then walk around on scrawny, weak legs. Not only can focusing on just a few muscle groups make you look unproportioned, it can also be unhealthy. Because the muscles' function is to provide stability and support for our skeleton, their overall alignment is a complex balance of tension and flexibility. If one side of the body is weaker than another side, postural imbalances leading to serious injuries can result.

There are two aspects to balance which must be considered in your training programme: strength and flexibility. Each muscle group needs to have both. How does this work?

Opposing pairs of muscles (front and back of the thigh, for example) act together. When a muscle group on one side of the body contracts, the opposite side lengthens. If it didn't then the movement of the bones would be limited. Look at the biceps and triceps in the front and back of your upper arm. When you bend your elbow, the biceps contract and the triceps lengthen in order for the arm to bend fully. If the triceps are not very flexible and the biceps are extra strong, then unnecessary strain and possible injury could occur from one forceful contraction.

Also, although several surrounding muscles may work together to perform a movement, it is usually the strongest one which does most of the work. If weaker muscles aren't strengthened along with others in the body, the stronger ones could end up compensating for them during certain actions. Then the weaker muscles don't end up supporting their joints properly. This can lead to misalignments in the spine and pelvis or excess shock and strain on the surrounding joints.

Muscle balance in the torso is especially important for a healthy back. Back pain is often due to weak muscles. Most women focus on abdominals and ignore the back and shoulder muscles which play an integral role in the posture. Strengthening the muscles in your upper back can help hunched shoulders, balance out a heavy lower body and make your waist look smaller.

The easiest way to make sure you are developing well-balanced muscles is to work all the muscle groups and vary your exercises periodically. It's also important to work in a full range of motion and call as many fibres in a muscle to work as possible. *The Squeeze* exercises in this book will provide you with a well-balanced muscle conditioning programme that will help improve your posture and enhance your shape.

Chapter 6

Common Questions About Weights

Common Questions About Weights

The only way seriously to improve your body shape is to use weights or some other form of resistance. Before you get frightened at the thought of pumping iron, let me reassure you that weights are not just for serious athletes. They can be used by men and women at any age. Physiotherapists commonly use weights on patients from 20 to 80 years old who are trying to strengthen their muscles after an injury. And you might be surprised to know that even ballet dancers train their lithe, sleek bodies with weights.

Weights are simple to use and you don't have to be highly coordinated to use them. You don't have to spend a lot of time learning complicated movements. Most importantly, they will give you quick results. Why?

Weights are a form of resistance. Resistance is simply an external force which makes your muscles work harder. When they work harder, they adapt by becoming stronger and firmer. The amount of resistance should be enough that it is a challenge, but not so hard that the muscle or surrounding joints are strained in trying to overcome the resistance.

Which Type of Resistance is Best?

Weights: Weights have been used by physical therapists for years. The problem is, most people wait until their muscles have weakened enough to allow an injury before they start using them.

The advantage of weights is that they allow you to manipulate the amount you use very precisely. If one muscle group is weak (the back of the upper arm, for example), you can use a lighter weight than you would when working a stronger muscle group (say, the front of the thigh). If a specific area in one muscle is weaker than other areas you can perform part of the same exercise with a light weight and progress to a heavier weight in the range of motion that is stronger. There are two types of weights you can train with: weight machines and free weights.

Weight Machines: These are the big steel contraptions you see in a gym. They are great for beginners since they have a designated seat and handles. They are easy to use because they automatically put you in proper positioning to perform an exercise. You don't have to remember specific exercises because the machine leads you through the desired movement. When you sit down, the handles will be positioned in a specific place (over your head, for example). You grab them and pull down (or push, depending on the exercise). This action targets the appropriate muscles for that particular machine. But because weight machines make you train in a specified position, there is a limited selection of exercises which can be performed on them.

Usually a machine will work just one muscle group so you have to use 6–12 machines to get a well-balanced workout. Unless you have the space in your home and money to purchase this much equipment, you'll have to join your local health club or leisure centre. Although you can buy a smaller 'multi gym', which is simply one piece of equipment with various bars and pulleys on it, it still takes up a lot of space and you'll end up spending hundreds of pounds to do the same exercises that you can do with £10–20 worth of small, portable, free weights.

Free Weights: These are individual weights, most commonly dumbbells, which you can hold in your hand. They can give you a much more flexible workout than weight machines because you can change the positions in which you do your exercises. By working the same muscle in a variety of planes, you target more fibres and work the muscle more thoroughly. Most weight machines isolate a muscle and work it alone before working another muscle. With free weights you can also work muscles in groups. As well, free weights call other muscles into action to help you balance the moving limb and stabilise the torso. Although you do have to learn which exercises to do, once you're familiar with them, free weights are better all round.

Elastic Bands and Rubber Tubing: These are another type of resistance tool. They don't look anything like weights but they work the same way. If you've never seen them before, they are colourful rubber strips or tubes. Some are simply giant versions of your everyday rubber band (big enough to wrap around both thighs). Others are long strips of plastic which you hold on each end and pull in different positions and directions. Others are more elaborate and consist of a tube with handles on the ends. No matter what their form, bands are a user-friendly alternative since they're light and compact.

Rubber resistance works on the principle that the elastic has a certain amount of tension. To stretch the band, your muscle must exert increasing levels of force to overcome the resistance. The bands usually come in different strengths. The more flexible they are, the less resistance on your muscles. They look flimsy, but studies have shown they can give your muscles an effective strength-training workout. One study found that after using Dynabands (a form of giant elastic band) three days a week to work the shoulders, upper arm and thighs, the average strength gains were 7–24 percent, depending on the muscle groups worked. Average strength gains from weight-lifting programmes are similar – 10–25 percent, depending on the muscle and weight used.

Elastic bands do have limitations. You can't work all muscle groups in all positions very easily. Many people find the hand grip required more uncomfortable than holding weights. To alleviate this discomfort you can wear training gloves for protection or use bands which have handles attached.

It's also more difficult to control the tension in a band. Because the range of tension sizes of the bands are limited, you may be forced to make a bigger jump than you might be ready for when progressing from one band to the next. With weights you can increase very gradually.

Body Weight: This is also a very effective form of resistance. You can add more or less resistance to an exercise by manipulating how much weight the limb you're working must support. For example, if you stand, then bend and straighten your leg in an exercise squat, your muscles will work much harder than if you were to bend and straighten your legs while lying down.

The only problem is that there is a limited range of exercises you can do with this form of resistance, so for some muscle groups, you do need to use weights or bands.

Visualisation and Concentration: These are methods of *mental focus* which can also help you increase the resistance to work a muscle more effectively. If you don't want to increase the amount of weight you use, you can increase the intensity of an exercise in your mind. You can visualise, or picture different images which will enhance the way you perform an exercise. Or you can concentrate and focus on specific aspects of a movement. By bringing your mind to your muscle in this way, you can really make the muscle work harder.

The Squeeze technique uses mental focus, free weights and occasionally body weight as its primary methods of resistance.

Should I Use Heavy or Light Weights?

Many women use light weights because they think they can tone their muscles without building them up. Using light weights when you *begin* a resistance training programme may be effective; your muscle may not be very strong at first, so this light weight is probably enough to fatigue it enough to build strength and some tone.

But if all you continue to do is lift a 1 lb (0.5 kg) weight, eventually your muscles will become accustomed to it and you'll stop forcing them to develop. The only way to keep your muscles challenged each time is to lift those light weights over and over and over and over… By increasing only the length of time you exercise, however, you will only improve your endurance. In order to improve your strength, you have to increase the *intensity* at

which you work. If you're trying to get firmer, you need to build strength rather than endurance.

Should I Lift Light Weights Many Times to Avoid Getting Bulky?

The tendency to 'bulk up' is largely genetic and females naturally have less muscle mass. So even if you want to get bulky, it's very difficult. You have to train with very heavy weights for hours a day.

The often quoted rule which says to use *heavier weights with lower repetitions* to build strength and bulk and to use *lighter weights with higher repetitions* to avoid increasing muscle mass really only applies to serious body-builders who use weights as heavy as 20 or 40 lb (9 or 18 kg), not the light weights of 1, 5 or 8 lb (0.5, 2, 3.5 kg) used by most women to avoid building bulk. You may build significantly less bulk by doing 15 repetitions with a 5 or 8 lb (2 or 3.5 kg) weight compared to three repetitions with a 50 lb (23 kg) weight. But the difference in bulk you'll gain from lifting 10 lb (4 kg) as opposed to 5 lb (2 kg) is negligible.

Exactly How Much Weight Should I Begin With?

▪ I would recommend starting with 2–5 lb (1–2 kg) dumbbells. When you buy weights, you may wish to start with one pair of 1 lb (0.5 kg) weights and one pair of 3 lb (1 kg) weights. You can start with one or two (hold both the weights in one hand). Then progress to 3 lb (1.5 kg). Then progress to 4 lb (2 kg) by holding a 3 lb (1.5 kg) and a 1 lb (0.5 kg) weight in your hand and so on.

▪ For safety reasons it's best to start with a light weight and work your way up. If you pick up a weight and feel strain in your joints right away, or if you can hardly move it, it's too heavy. If you can swing the weight around very easily, it's probably too light.

- For strength and toning, if you feel fatigued from doing 8–15 repetitions of one set of exercises, then whatever weight you are using is appropriate. If you feel as though you could keep going, you should increase the weight.

- Although I do recommend that you use a fairly heavy weight, do be aware that if you start out with too much weight you can overstress the joint. If you're unsure, refer back to page 46.

- Remember, too, that different muscle groups are stronger than others. You may be able to use quite heavy weights for your biceps (upper inner arms) and deltoids (shoulders), but need very light ones for your triceps (backs of the upper arm) or trapezius (upper back).

How Many Repetitions of an Exercise Should I Do?

I remember a Gary Larson 'Far Side' cartoon captioned 'Aerobics in hell'. The characters were doing leg lifts and the devil was shouting, 'One million and one, one million and two...' While the norm used to be that everyone prolonged 'the burn', the good news is that you shouldn't. Rather than go for precise numbers, you can go by the way you feel. But if you are training for strength, then you want to make sure that your muscles feel fatigued within 30–90 seconds of performing an exercise. Studies have shown that working a specific muscle any longer than this means you focus more on developing endurance. For most people, this is best accomplished using

about 75 percent of the maximum force a muscle can exert, then doing 8–12 repetitions of an exercise. The exercise should be done slowly, rather than fast.

At the end of each set of repetitions, you should feel a slight discomfort. This is normal muscular fatigue which shows that your muscles are being challenged to exert enough force that they tire out. Reaching this state is what will elicit adaptations from the muscle fibres.

If you feel nothing at the end of a set of exercises, chances are you haven't challenged the muscles enough and you will only maintain, not improve upon, your current levels of strength and tone.

How Many Sets Should I Do?

One set is a group of repetitions. So if you do 12 repetitions, for example, you have performed 'one set' of an exercise. If you've been lifting weights, you're probably familiar with the traditional training formula: three sets of 8–12 repetitions each. Some body-builders may do five sets or more of each exercise.

New research shows that three sets may be a waste of time if your only concern is to build strength or muscle mass. You can experience almost the same increase in strength from doing *one set* of 8–12 reps as from doing *two or three*. Eighty percent of the physical gains you will achieve from doing three sets is achieved by doing one set only.

This seems odd – surely the more you do, the stronger you'll get? Actually, as I've emphasised all along with *The Squeeze* technique, the key is *quality*, not quantity. The principle of resistance training is that you challenge a muscle to work harder than it normally does. As long as you push the muscle to a certain intensity, it doesn't matter much how often you do so. It will continue to remain or grow strong enough to handle this amount of force.

Common Questions About Weights

This aspect of training also applies to other types of fitness. If you have been working out four or five days a week to increase your stamina and overall fitness level, you can actually maintain your current fitness level even if you decrease the number of days you exercise. The key is to exercise at a high intensity on the two or three days that you do work out. Less is more.

The 'one set' programme is great news for people with not much time or motivation. But if you really enjoy the meditative aspect of resistance training, doing up to a total of three sets will also help you burn more calories and, depending upon the order and intensity of the exercises, you can also gain a cardiovascular benefit, as you would walking or cycling. You will achieve slightly more strength gains and the extra effort will also aid in fat loss.

How Fast Should I Move During These Exercises?

There is no cut and dried rule with regards to speed. Going slower generally makes you work a little harder. Unless otherwise indicated, you should aim to move very slowly through each phase of the movement. For example, if you are pushing your arms over your head, aim to push up for the count of two (one, two). Then hold the position for a second to stop the momentum and focus on control. Then lower slowly to the count of two, or even four, again (one, two). Concentrate on going a little slower during the return phase. Consciously resist the reflex to swing back, or drop down to your starting position.

Some athletes lift very heavy weights very quickly. This is usually to train for more power and agility in their sport. The average exerciser may find this type of training too intense.

Circuit Training: Another form of resistance training is *circuit training* in which participants move quickly from one weight exercise to another. The weights used are generally quite light and this type of workout is an attempt to combine an aerobic cardiovascular workout with a strength training one. It is an invigorating workout but it's very tough. It's not easy for a beginner to push themselves this hard. I recommend that you do circuit training under professional supervision at a health club. The faster you move through exercises, the less time you have to monitor your technique or develop an inner focus on what you're doing and feeling. Lack of concentration and control means a greater risk of injury.

The Squeeze technique will teach you how to execute an exercise properly. By practising it you can train your body to get in the habit of good execution. When you have reached this stage, you'll be better equipped to move through the intense exercises at a faster pace in a circuit training class.

How Often Should I Do Resistance Training?

If finding the time to work out is a major problem, here's the good news: experts actually advise *against* working your muscles too often. Whereas you can do aerobic exercise daily, performing resistance exercises with bands and weights exhausts your muscles so much that they need time to recover. Because muscle conditioning work is very intense, you should not do these exercises every day. This is not because I have developed a miracle method where you sit on your bum and squeeze it to watch the inches fall off! (This technique, which had had great claims made for it in the past, has been shown to be physiologically impossible.)

But the less frequently you pump iron, the stronger and more toned you'll become. So for best results lift weights every other day. Rest is good, so do not feel guilty for not exercising as long as you are doing these exercises two or three days a week (but with approximately 48 hours in between sessions). You should also do aerobic, whole body exercise at least two or three times a week.

There are some people who do perform resistance exercises every day. This is OK as long as you are working different muscle groups on consecutive days. Typically, body-builders may train their biceps and triceps on Monday, their chest and quadriceps on Tuesday, their lower body and back on Wednesday and biceps and triceps on Thursday, for example. Usually instead of doing just one exercise per muscle group, they will do several different moves, training the same muscle at several different angles, in order to target the widest range of muscle fibres. This is known as 'blasting' a muscle. If you're motivated to do this – and more importantly, *keep it up* – this is fine. But you'll see more benefits if you do a smaller amount of exercise over a long period of time, rather than a lot of exercise for a very short period.

Because of my teaching schedule, I usually lift weights on Mondays and Thursday. When I can, I also do them on Saturdays, although this varies from week to week. I work all my muscle groups, doing one set of 12 repetitions in one workout. I do the same exercises for a three- to four-week period, then vary the exercises slightly after each period.

If I Stop Exercising Will my Muscles Turn to Fat?

Contrary to popular belief, a muscle will not turn into fat. If it is unused for a period – whilst in a plaster cast, for example – muscle tissue may be lost and fat tissue may be increased, but one will not turn into the other. If you have been lifting weights and then stop, gains in performance and strength will be noticeably lost after three to four weeks. You may notice the muscle getting more flabby, but the area won't automatically get fat.

Is It OK to Use Weights During Aerobic Activities?

The 'heavy hands' approach of using 1–2 lb (0.5–1 kg) weights to burn more calories when you are doing aerobics (like in 'New Body' classes, walking, running, or stepping) is futile. Study after study has shown that these weights do not increase the intensity of your workout: you don't burn more calories. Sometimes you burn even fewer than you would doing the aerobic activity without, because the movement is usually slowed down in order to control the speed of the weights and exercise technique. There's also a high risk of straining the shoulder and elbow joints. Heavier weights will burn more calories but exponentially increase the injury risk. Instead, experts recommend that you drop the iron and run, step or walk *faster or longer* to fire up your metabolism.

How Long Do I Have to Keep Lifting Weights?

Exercise is based on controlled stress to the body. By forcing your muscles to work harder than normal, they will adapt by becoming stronger. If you stop challenging them, they will cease to improve further. If you stop altogether, eventually you will return to your former unfit state. But how long that takes depends on how fit you were and how long you had been fit to begin with.

If you are currently lifting weights three times a week, once you reach a desired level of strength, to maintain it studies suggest that all you need to do is resistance exercises once or twice per week. The key is to keep the intensity up – *work hard* – when you do train.

Common Questions About Weights

Tips

If you constantly use a light weight and do the same exercises without varying them, your muscles will not be forced to improve. In an effort to be efficient with energy use, they will quickly adapt, learning to recruit the minimum number of muscle fibres possible. For maximum tone you want to train as many of the fibres within a muscle as possible.

The most efficient way to do this is to overload a muscle, to aim for maximum contraction. This is most easily done by simply increasing the amount of resistance and therefore the amount of force required from a muscle.

But there are also other ways to refine your technique before you actually increase the weight. In fact, before progressing on to a heavier weight, it is better to perfect your execution at your current level so that you develop control as well as strength.

Work Slowly: Moving slowly during any conditioning exercise is crucial. Decreasing the speed allows more time for the brain to send signals to activate more muscle fibres so there is a greater potential for the muscle to work harder. You also have more time to think and monitor all aspects of the movement. In *The Squeeze* technique I will show you how to make slow, precise movements.

That's not to say that fast, explosive movements are incorrect. Many sports require that you be able to move in this way, but the average exerciser simply looking to improve basic strength and muscle tone should stick to slow movements.

Generally, aim to move the weight to the count of two, pause for a second, then return the weight to starting position even slower to the count of four. Avoid using momentum to activate the movement.

Move Through a Full Range of Motion: Working through a full range of motion means moving a joint as far as the muscle you are working allows it to bend and straighten.

Experiment with a biceps curl. Bend your elbow, bringing your fist up to your shoulder, then straighten the elbow completely. This is the full range of motion for the biceps muscle. If you were to bend your elbow to 90 degrees and then lift your fist up and down a little way without bending or straightening all the way, you would be working in a limited range of motion. This means you would only be working a small part of the muscle and this can lead to muscle imbalances.

Contract Your Muscles Correctly: There are several ways for a muscle to contract. When you move your body through an exercise, the muscle first shortens as it develops tension and overcomes the resistance. This phase, called the *concentric* phase, as mentioned earlier, is the main part of the contraction, where you develop power and strength. In an abdominal curl the concentric phase is when you bring your ribs towards your hips. The return phase of the movement when the muscle lengthens as it overcomes the resistance is called the *eccentric* contraction. The eccentric phase is usually aided by gravity such as when you lower your shoulders to the floor during an abdominal curl. There is less effort required during the return phase of a move so the muscle works less.

Many people hurry through this phase so they can start the next repetition. But it is important to develop strength in both phases of the action. So concentrate on moving more slowly to make the muscle work harder during this part of the movement.

You may have heard of another type of contraction known as the *isometric squeeze*. This is a way of working within a limited range of motions. There are several exercise programmes, including Callanetics and the Lotte Berk method, which rely on lots of isometric exercises: tiny squeezing movements. While you can gain some strength in this way, overall it is not a balanced or effective way of overloading a muscle. It's fine to include these type of moves within a well-balanced programme of exercises which work the muscles through their full range of motion, but not to do them exclusively. If you did *only* these type of movements, you could develop muscle imbalances leading to injury.

Breathe Well: You will also experience more power in your moves by breathing correctly. Breathing slowly helps you relax and a relaxed muscle can contract more powerfully than a tensed one. Try lifting a weight or pushing someone away when you're being tickled, for example. It's very hard to muster up any strength at all because the muscles become tense.

Going slowly and breathing fully will help bring you from a totally relaxed state to a contracted state. Aim to exhale on the effort, that is, when you move the weight. Then inhale on the return, when you bring the weight back to the starting position.

Resistance Training Dos and Don'ts

▨ Avoid locking the joints, especially the elbows and knees.

▨ If you're using bands, they should be stretched, rather than slack, throughout the whole exercise.

▨ If you cannot stretch the band through the full range of motion of an exercise, go for a lighter resistance.

▨ Perform the exercises slowly so you use muscular control, rather than momentum.

▨ Breathe evenly. Exhale when you push or pull the weight. Inhale when you return to the starting position.

▨ During side leg lifts, hold the weight or wrap a band above the knee. Many people wrap bands around the ankles for inner and outer thigh exercises. Since the downward pull of the foot from the resistance counteracts with the upward pull of the thigh movement, there can be excessive tension on the knee.

▨ Your *muscles* should feel fatigued from the exercises. But if you feel pain in your *joints*, stop.

▨ When holding a weight or elastic band, your wrist should be kept straight in line with the forearm, rather than flexed.

Precautions

Hypertensives have traditionally been warned off strength training since lifting weights can raise your blood pressure. In fact, done properly, strength training will not *adversely* affect your blood pressure and over the long term can actually help decrease it. If you do have high blood pressure it is especially important to breathe throughout each exercise and avoid any isometric moves (where you hold a position and squeeze).

Arthritis has also been shown to be helped through resistance training. But with any serious medical condition, please get a doctor's approval and also see a chartered physiotherapist if necessary before exercising.

Get Squeezing

Weight lifting is the only exercise method that can transform your body. The fact is, as we age, we lose muscle mass. This is what causes the sags, the droops and the lowered metabolism which makes us gain weight more easily. If you start doing resistance training now, you won't necessarily be building your muscles up, you'll be maintaining what you have. Hollywood stars, whose bodies are their business, know that the key to looking young is resistance training. That's why you'll find that everyone, from Madonna and Demi Moore to Jane Fonda and even older stars, trains regularly with weights.

But weights are only part of the solution. You have to know how to use them. Now I will introduce you to *The Squeeze* technique.

Chapter 7

Feel, Focus, Squeeze, Control

Feel, Focus, Squeeze, Control

The *Squeeze* technique helps you focus in to work out. This will change the way you exercise. But be aware that it's not always easy to concentrate when you exercise. Sometimes it's easier to tune out. Sometimes you do it without even realising it. You might exercise in a group situation and look at the instructor or people around you. Or when exercising at home you may become engrossed in a TV show or conversation. If you exercise to music, you can easily lose yourself in the melody. Even just counting down your repetitions in an exercise to help you get through to the finish is distracting.

But sometimes the distraction is more mental. If you're very competitive you might focus on the speed or on your moves, rather than on the technique. Or if you're angry, you may exercise to release your frustration. If you feel fat, your main stimulus when you work out might be the desire to sweat and feel skinnier. You can start out focused, but then lose it towards the end of a set of exercises. This causes you to rush through the last few or lose the intensity as you lose interest.

Consider the following scenario.

It's six o'clock. You've been stuck in traffic. You have people coming round at eight. You're in a hurry but need to fit in some exercise since you've been putting it off all week. You grab your clothes, run to the gym and jump into a class that has already started. Or you pull on some trainers and put on a fitness video. While you follow it you think of what you're going to wear, try to remember what it was you've forgotten to do and look around the room, noting that after a shower, makeup and phone calls to return, you need to quickly tidy up. You finish the workout and get back to work.

No matter how you approached your workout, there's no doubt that you will feel better for having exercised. You burned calories, worked your muscles and accomplished one of the things on your list. It's positive that you did it at all. Sometimes you are distracted and that can't be avoided. Sometimes disassociating yourself can even help motivate you if you're apt to give up. If you exercise often, it can be a way to alleviate boredom. Or you may be able to solve a few work or personal problems by thinking about then when you work out.

But avoid letting distraction be your main approach to exercise. You simply won't get the physical and mental benefits that you could if you focused more instead. Since you've managed to slot in time for yourself, why not make the most of it? As I mentioned in Chapter 2, concentrating on one thing can have a meditative, relaxing effect. So if you focus on the task at hand, your movement and all the feelings associated with it, you'll give your mind a break, allowing you to unwind. Rather than just finish the workout relieved that you did it, you will feel mentally refreshed and re-energised for the rest of the day.

The difference between mindlessly going through the motions or luxuriating in the process of your body's movement is your ability to go within, to feel and focus. It's the act of centring yourself.

Centring Yourself

By becoming more observant you'll synchronise your mind and body. By becoming more aware you'll develop a deeper understanding of how to move.

Imagine that you are at a friend's house. You walk to the kitchen and pass another room on the way. You could ignore it altogether. You could glance at it and notice a few obvious details. Or you could stop and really look at what's inside. How much detail you see is up to you. You could see furniture and notice the colour and size. You could see pictures and notice who's in them. You may even start to take this information and process it. Is that man in the picture your friend's brother? Is this the pillow she told you she bought while on holiday? The more you notice, the more you get to know that room and that person. This sticks in your memory so that the next time you are there you notice even more and the things you are already familiar with become natural.

The same process happens when you focus in and practise *The Squeeze*. As you focus, you learn more about how your body responds and feels and moves. And the more you are aware, the more you can use your knowledge to perfect your exercise technique.

The basis of *The Squeeze* technique is to *feel, focus, squeeze* and *control*. To concentrate effectively you must first develop an overall awareness of your body. When you *feel*, you can then *focus* and direct your attention to your alignment, your *squeeze* or whatever needs attending to. This process gives you the *control* to get the most out of your movement.

The Four Golden Principles of *The Squeeze* Technique

Feel: This is the starting phase to help you concentrate and block out any distractions. As you begin to exercise, be aware of how you feel – your legs, your arms, your torso, your neck. Don't just be aware of your pain threshold – with *The Squeeze* you are delving deeper.

Be aware of your positioning. Are you balanced, or do you feel a bit of tension somewhere in your body which is causing you to lean forward or twist or slump? Be aware of your energy output. Feel the movement. In looking *out*, you distance yourself from your body. I want you to get closer by looking *in*.

Being aware of how all the relevant parts of your body feel means you're less likely to get injured. You can also fine-tune your moves to make them even more effective. You can change the tension of a stretch, or the angle of a limb if you feel too much stress. You can up the force you exert or decrease the intensity to make the exercise harder or easier.

Focus: Shift your focus according to where it's needed. If you feel unbalanced, shift your attention to your feet and move them so that you have a more stable base of support. If you feel pain in your leg, zoom to the cause of the pain and modify your move to reduce it.

To analyse a muscle contraction, consider: Is my muscle contracting fully? Am I working in a full range?

To monitor your joint action, determine: Is my knee twisting? Is my back leaning at a safe angle?

Feel, Focus, Squeeze, Control

To assess your body alignment, spot check: Are my ribs held high? Is my pelvis tilted?

To determine your perceived exertion, judge how you feel: Is this weight too heavy so that I feel strain in my joint? Should I slow down so that I rely less on momentum and more on muscular control?

In each of *The Squeeze* exercises, I will show you how to focus on the most essential parts of your body to execute a mindful movement. Every exercise has a few key areas which can be unduly stressed. I will give you precise pointers to check in each position.

Squeeze: The final stop in your focusing should be at the core of the exercise itself, the muscle and its movement. Most fitness teachers tend to emphasise the performance of the exercise. During abdominals they may tell you to press your back to the floor, tilt your pelvis or lift up. While these points are important, they fail to bring your mind to the centre of the move – in this case, the abdominal muscles.

Concentrating on extraneous aspects instead of the muscle contracting puts your focus elsewhere. You may achieve a weaker contraction than if you were to concentrate and squeeze the muscle more. Channelling your mental energy will translate into more physical energy. Because you are working from a relaxed state, when you finally bring your mind to your muscle you will be able to contract it with more power than if you were distracted. You will activate more muscle fibres and work the muscle more thoroughly. You will increase the intensity of your exercise. You will be putting more energy into it, but in a gentle way. You will definitely feel the difference.

As I mentioned early in the book, this is not only a difference in physical sensation, but also in your perspective. Remember it is the muscles which cause your body to move, not the other way around. By focusing on the core of an action you will have more control.

Control: This inner focus is a tool to enhance the way you perform *specific* exercises.

If you were to apply *The Squeeze* technique to whole body activities, like running, jumping and kicking, you'd be overanalytical about everything involved. It would slow you down and break up the synchronisation of muscle activities which make the movement. If you were trying to perfect a tennis serve, for example, it would be impossible to feel everything happening at every instant of the motion. Moreover, it would be hard to modify anything you might detect. Momentum, which *The Squeeze* aims to diminish in individual exercises, is actually an integral aspect of whole body activities. If you broke a ballet leap down into a number of minute points, the action simply could not occur. Therefore, during whole body activities, focus your attention on one predetermined thing only: the angle of your foot when you kick a soccer ball, for example, or the follow through when hitting a backhand. You are still focusing inwards, but in a different way.

Individual exercises rely on muscular control more than momentum. So here you can slow things down without affecting the exercise. This means you have time to analyse and make adjustments.

With *The Squeeze* technique I want to take you one step further. Once you've listened, evaluated and reacted to your body signals, I want you to not only feel the body part alone, but also feel it as part of the whole movement. I want you to feel the synchronisation of your body: the bones, the muscles, the joints and how everything flows together. I want you to move as one and luxuriate in the feeling. This is when your exercise will feel effortless. This is control.

Chapter 8

The Squeeze Technique

The Squeeze Technique

You've learned about your mind, muscles and movement. Now you can put your knowledge into practice. The aim of *The Squeeze* technique is to feel and control each movement.

The following exercises are the basic moves to begin your programme. Many of these exercises may look familiar. Instead of skipping them, stop and consider each one carefully. Perfect your technique. You will experience even the simplest exercise in a totally new way. You may have been doing basic abdominal exercises or leg lifts for years, but chances are you have done them without a full awareness of exact body positioning, limb alignment and focus. There is a difference between doing an exercise mindlessly and doing an exercise with a thorough understanding of its perfect execution.

The Squeeze technique gives you an in-depth analysis of each exercise. I first lead you through the position from start to finish. Then I show the body parts on which to focus in order to get the most benefit. You will learn exactly how your body should align during each move. Pay attention to all the sensations. Then concentrate on the action of the muscle – execute the squeeze. Finally, perform the move with effortless control.

Of course, you don't have to be hyper-analytical about every single movement. You can still benefit, no matter how strong your focus. Whether you're really concentrating or just aimlessly moving around, you are exercising, after all. But by using *The Squeeze* technique you can work better. You can maximise the quality of your movement to expend less effort and less time to get better results.

The Basic Exercises

The basic exercises I have given you generally isolate one major muscle. This means that the movement is fairly simple – reaching up or down or pushing the leg forwards and backwards, for example. In some cases, however, the move may be quite straight-forward, but more than one muscle will be worked. This is because surrounding muscles tend to work together to perform an action.

Use these exercises to perfect your technique and develop control. You will become stronger and develop more muscle tone. When you can sufficiently perform these exercises with control and strength, you can then move on to the more challenging *Squeeze* exercises. I have marked these with three stars.

Advanced *Squeeze* Exercises

The advanced *Squeeze* exercises are multi-muscle moves. This means that they don't just target one muscle, but several muscle groups are integrated into one motion. So instead of doing an arm movement to work just the deltoids, an advanced exercise might include work on the trapezius, deltoids and pectorals.

Once you've developed a base level of strength and coordination and the ability to isolate and focus on each particular muscle, then you can graduate to more sophisticated movements. By practising more coordinated movements you can improve the muscles' ability to respond to brain signals and the grace and precision such movements require will improve your overall coordination. They will also vary the stimuli on your body, as you are no longer doing the same exercise time after time.

Become proficient with the basic exercises first, so you develop a good base level of strength and control. Then add the advanced exercises to your routine, first without weights, then with them once you feel fitter.

I have provided the following information for each exercise:

- muscles worked;
- the positioning for each phase of the movement;
- special emphasis on various body parts so you can monitor your alignment;
- safety tips to avoid straining the body;
- a mental image to help you visualise and understand the action;
- modifications so you work harder/easier depending on how you feel;
- directions on how to squeeze during the exercise.

The exercises are grouped by body parts. In some cases I have provided several different exercises that target the same muscle groups. It will be best to go through each exercise and to determine which ones you prefer.

You will not need to do every exercise every time you work out. Later, in Chapter 12, I will give you a specialised routine to follow. When an exercise becomes easy, or when you feel as though you need some diversity, then you can substitute a different exercise to work the same muscle group. As I mentioned earlier, it is better to keep variety in your workout. You'll work the muscles more thoroughly and will be less likely to get bored.

Here are the points to remember:

- Feel, focus, squeeze and control.
- Move slowly for better awareness.
- Focus on internal sensations. If you are distracted, breathe deeply and gently shift your focus back.
- Feel the level of tension during all phases of the movement, from start to finish.
- Make your movement effortless.
- Pause after each phase of a movement.

You are now ready to try out the exercises. After following the exercise programme, you will notice an improvement in your body shape, your posture and the way you walk. You will also be able to incorporate other fitness activities such as sports and dance into your lifestyle. By practising these *Squeeze* exercises you will become more and more coordinated. No matter what your age or fitness level now, you can become the natural athlete you never thought you could be. This could open up a whole new world of experience to you. Even if you have no desire to start playing tennis or taking ballet lessons now, if you were to try after this mind–body training, you might discover you love it – and, more importantly, add a new fun physical activity to your repertoire. This means fewer repetitive exercise sessions, more diversity and a chance to develop a whole new side of yourself.

Chapter 9

The Squeeze Exercises – Lower Body

Legs and Buttocks

The Squeeze Exercises – Lower Body

Now it is time to put your mind into your muscle and fine-tune your movements. Study each move for a thorough understanding of how the muscles you are working function. Listen to how each body part feels and adjust yourself accordingly. Go through each exercise at least once without using added weight, just to familiarise yourself with the natural stresses involved before you add additional resistance. Then refer back to page 46 to determine how much weight you should start with and go to Chapter 12 to schedule an exercise routine.

I provide you with the following information for each exercise:

Exercise Name

I have chosen exercise names which I feel best depict the move. You may know the same exercise by a different name.

Muscles Worked

If you want to impress your friends, memorise the Latin names for all the skeletal muscles! Since most exercises work several muscles in different ways, I will list just the primary muscles in action.

Use the names to refer back to the muscle illustrations on pages 28–35 so you can see exactly where the muscles lie on a body part. By seeing where the end points of a muscle group are connected and the direction in which the muscle fibres run, you can better understand the movement which a muscle performs. This will help develop your inner focus so you can work your body more effectively.

Position

I have broken down each exercise into a starting and ending position. For the advanced *Squeeze* exercises, or those whose action is not clearly depicted visually, I have added more transitional positions. These sections simply give you the basic positioning and action.

I have indicated the breathing pattern to follow during the move as well and also made special notes for particular body parts (hips, arms, back, neck, etc.). These alignment tips will help you hold everything in its right place. By knowing exactly what all key areas should do, you will have much more control in an exercise.

Safety Tip

Since understanding an exercise means not only knowing what to do, but what *not* to do, I have alerted you to potential stresses to avoid during an exercise.

■ **Mental Image**

In order to enhance the sensation of the action, I have provided a mental image which you can visualise as you move. This is often a quick way to instinctively hold yourself and move in the correct position.

■ **Squeeze**

Once you are comfortable with the technique and alignment required for a move, you can shift your inner focus back to the main muscle groups you are working. I will tell you where to concentrate the tension to execute a movement. Remember that by consciously bringing your mind to your muscle you can train it to work more effectively. As I mentioned earlier, you need to focus in on the muscle and contract it to cause the movement. For example, to get the full benefit of the mind–body connection, you need to squeeze your abdominal muscles in order to move your torso, rather than move your body in order to work the abdominals. *The Squeeze* is a subtle shift in perspective to bring you to the core of the action.

■ **Modification**

I will give you an 'easy' or 'hard' modification of the exercise. This is usually just a shift in position to add more or less resistance. If an exercise is too hard, you can also decrease your weight to make it easier. If you want more of a challenge, increase the resistance in some way, either by increasing the weight or intensifying your mental focus. But also remember that you will want to work at different intensities on different days. Even if you are very fit, if you are tired one day, or simply want to vary the move a bit, feel free to choose the easier version.

■ **Fit Fact**

I will share something fascinating with you about the body part you're working. The human body is a wondrous thing!

Squat

The Squeeze: At the lowest point of the squat, focus on your buttocks and squeeze them tightly to push back up to a standing position.

Muscles worked: quadriceps, hamstrings, gluteus maximus

Mental Image
Imagine that you are about to sit in a chair. Your buttocks reach out behind you to find the seat.

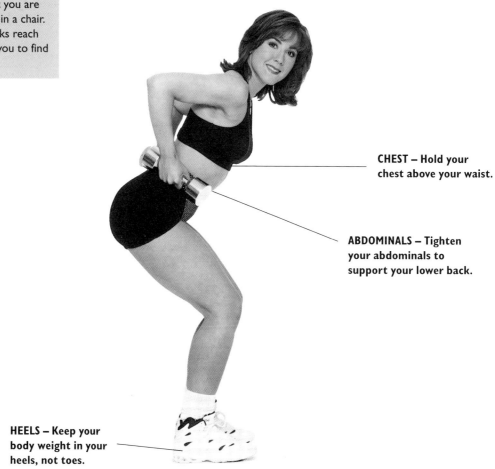

CHEST – Hold your chest above your waist.

ABDOMINALS – Tighten your abdominals to support your lower back.

HEELS – Keep your body weight in your heels, not toes.

Position 1. Stand tall with your feet shoulder width apart. Hold your weights on your hips or shoulders. With a straight back, lean at a slight angle forwards.

Safety Tip
If you feel any stress in your knees, push your hips farther out at the back as you lower. You should be able to lift your toes up in your shoes since your body weight is in your heels. If your back hurts, make sure that you are lowering your hips rather than bending back and forth at the waist.

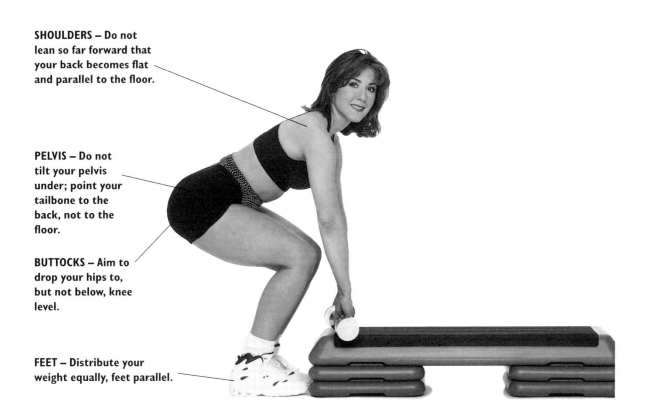

SHOULDERS – Do not lean so far forward that your back becomes flat and parallel to the floor.

PELVIS – Do not tilt your pelvis under; point your tailbone to the back, not to the floor.

BUTTOCKS – Aim to drop your hips to, but not below, knee level.

FEET – Distribute your weight equally, feet parallel.

Position 2. As you exhale, push your hips out behind you and lower your buttocks. Allow your hands to fall down in front as you lower your body. Make sure you do not push your knees forward. They should stay above your ankles (not toes) at all times. Inhale and straighten up.

Modification
If your back hurts, lift your shoulders higher as you lower. But make sure that you do keep your body weight in your heels. Instead of squeezing tightly at the low end of the squat, squeeze at the top when you return to standing.

Squat Kick

The Squeeze: Concentrate on squeezing the buttocks, especially as you lower into the squat and as you bring your lifted leg back down.

Muscles worked: gluteals, quadriceps, adductors

Mental Image
Imagine you are a ballet dancer and move as slowly as possible as you lift *and* as you lower.

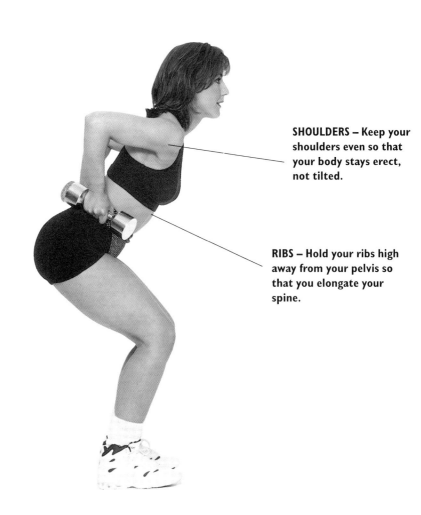

SHOULDERS – Keep your shoulders even so that your body stays erect, not tilted.

RIBS – Hold your ribs high away from your pelvis so that you elongate your spine.

Position 1. Stand with your feet parallel, shoulder width apart. Keep your body weight in your heels. Tighten your abdominals and with a straight back, lean at a slight angle forwards. Lower your hips as you push them out behind so you are in a basic squat position. Do not tilt your pelvis forward. Hold the weights on your hips.

Safety Tip
At each different stage of this exercise, hold your body still for one second so that you perform this exercise with control and maintain perfect alignment throughout.

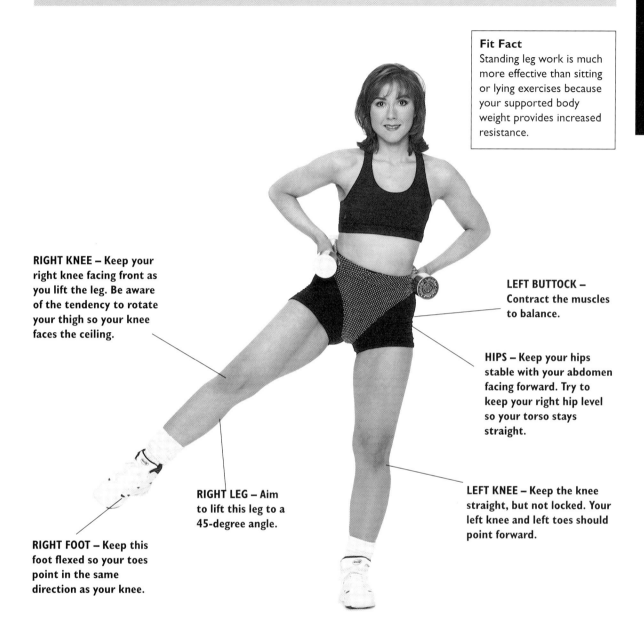

RIGHT KNEE – Keep your right knee facing front as you lift the leg. Be aware of the tendency to rotate your thigh so your knee faces the ceiling.

LEFT BUTTOCK – Contract the muscles to balance.

HIPS – Keep your hips stable with your abdomen facing forward. Try to keep your right hip level so your torso stays straight.

RIGHT LEG – Aim to lift this leg to a 45-degree angle.

LEFT KNEE – Keep the knee straight, but not locked. Your left knee and left toes should point forward.

RIGHT FOOT – Keep this foot flexed so your toes point in the same direction as your knee.

Position 2. With your body weight still in your heels, exhale, squeeze your buttocks and straighten your legs while you kick your right leg out to the side. Hold for a second, then inhale and slowly lower your leg and return to the squat in position 1. Check your alignment, then squeeze and lift the other leg.

Squat Kick ***Advanced Exercise

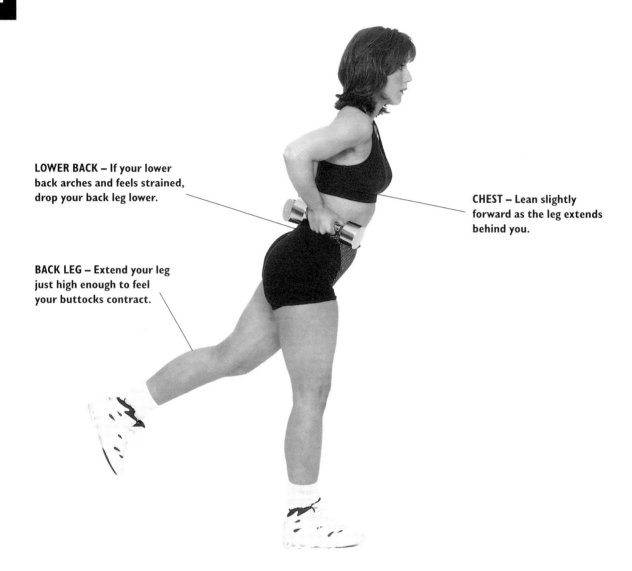

LOWER BACK – If your lower back arches and feels strained, drop your back leg lower.

CHEST – Lean slightly forward as the leg extends behind you.

BACK LEG – Extend your leg just high enough to feel your buttocks contract.

Position 3. After you have completed a squat and kick to each side, inhale and squat again, then exhale and straighten as you kick each leg behind you.

Modification
Once you can hold this position comfortably, for a more advanced muscle-toning move you can lift with your knee facing front, then, when you have reached a 45-degree angle, rotate your thigh so your knee faces up.

The Squeeze: Squeeze the back of your thigh, especially as you lower your foot.

Muscles worked: hamstring group

Fit Fact
The hamstrings are most active when you walk or run. Since the front of the thigh tends to be stronger, keep the hamstrings toned as well.

Mental Image
Pretend that your back foot is stuck with sticky glue onto the floor. As you bend your knee, feel your foot pulling away to stretch the glue.

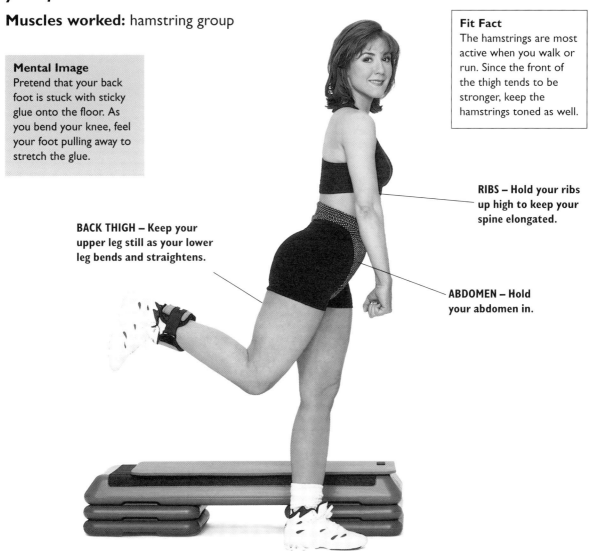

RIBS – Hold your ribs up high to keep your spine elongated.

BACK THIGH – Keep your upper leg still as your lower leg bends and straightens.

ABDOMEN – Hold your abdomen in.

Position 1. Put an ankle weight on, or place a light weight inside your sock. Extend your right leg straight behind you so your right foot is about 6 inches (15 cm) behind your left heel.

Position 2. Contract your buttocks and your abdominals to stabilise your upper thigh. Then exhale and slowly bend your back knee and bring your heel to the back of your thigh. Hold for a second, then inhale and slowly straighten your leg by dropping the foot down. Repeat, then switch legs.

Safety Tip
If your back hurts, make sure that you are not arching it as you lift your foot.

Leg Reach

The Squeeze: When you reach out, squeeze your buttocks. When you pull in, squeeze the inside of the upper thigh.

Muscles worked: inner thighs, gluteus medius and minimus, sartorius

Mental Image
Pretend there is a magnet on the standing inner thigh. Feel the inner thigh of the extended leg contracting as it is drawn to the supporting leg.

Fit Fact
Most activities we do tend to focus on the front and back of the thigh (walking, running, stepping, cycling). The outer and inner thigh muscles are used less, except during activities such as skiing and skating.

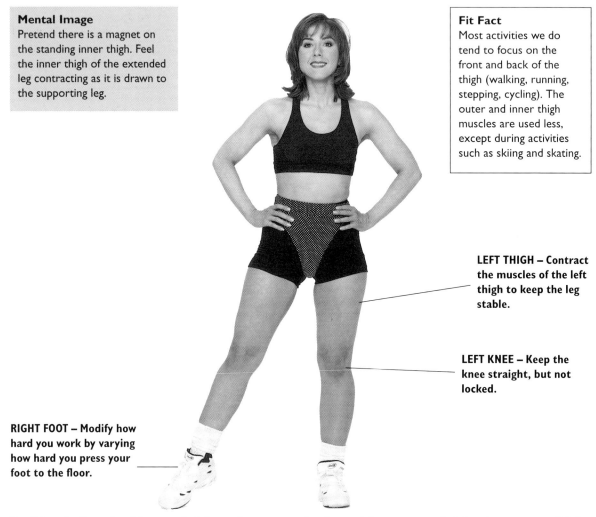

LEFT THIGH – Contract the muscles of the left thigh to keep the leg stable.

LEFT KNEE – Keep the knee straight, but not locked.

RIGHT FOOT – Modify how hard you work by varying how hard you press your foot to the floor.

Position 1. Stand with your left knee bent, your body weight on your left heel, not toes. Make sure your left knee and toes are facing out in the same direction. Inhale and extend your right leg out to the side as far as you can. Then exhale and push your foot into the floor and drag your right thigh to the left leg, then straighten both. Repeat, alternating legs.

Modification.
This exercise concentrates primarily on the inner thighs, with some resistance to work the buttocks and outer thighs. To target the outer thighs more, attach an ankle weight so that you have to reach out through more resistance.

Safety Tip
If you feel any strain in your knee, turn your thigh out so that you lead with your heel rather than with the side of your foot.

Calf Raise

The Squeeze: Move slowly as you lift so you can feel the calf contracting. Don't focus on pushing with your toes, concentrate and squeeze the calf.

Muscles worked: gastrocnemius, soleus

Mental Image
Pretend you are a tree reaching toward the sun as you lift.

Fit Fact
Strong calves can provide stability for the knee and ankle joints. Make sure you also stretch these muscles to help maintain balance in your lower leg.

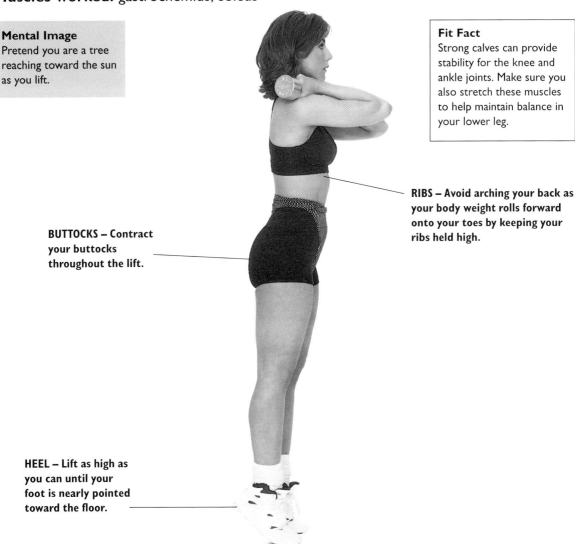

RIBS – Avoid arching your back as your body weight rolls forward onto your toes by keeping your ribs held high.

BUTTOCKS – Contract your buttocks throughout the lift.

HEEL – Lift as high as you can until your foot is nearly pointed toward the floor.

Position 1. Stand with your feet parallel, hip width apart. Hold your weights on your shoulders.

Position 2. As you exhale, lift your body up by pushing onto the balls of your feet as high as you can. Keep your balance by positioning your body weight on your big and second toe. Inhale as you lower, then repeat.

Modification
Vary the direction in which your foot is turned. Turn the toes out or in. Then try the same move with your knee bent to target other muscles in the calf.

71

Inner Thigh Tightener *** Advanced Exercise

The Squeeze: Feel the stretch in your inner thighs when you open your legs, then focus on squeezing them together as tightly as possible.

Muscles worked: inner thigh group, quadriceps, hamstrings, gluteals

Mental Image
Pretend you have a cannonball attached to the outer leg as you pull it in.

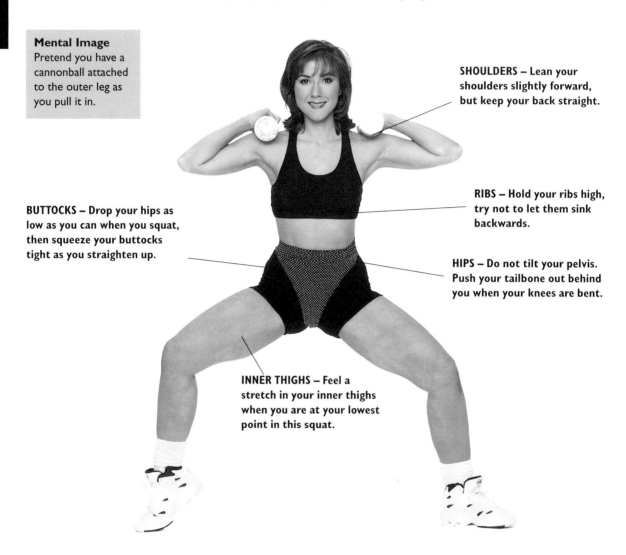

SHOULDERS – Lean your shoulders slightly forward, but keep your back straight.

RIBS – Hold your ribs high, try not to let them sink backwards.

BUTTOCKS – Drop your hips as low as you can when you squat, then squeeze your buttocks tight as you straighten up.

HIPS – Do not tilt your pelvis. Push your tailbone out behind you when your knees are bent.

INNER THIGHS – Feel a stretch in your inner thighs when you are at your lowest point in this squat.

Position 1. Hold your weights on your shoulders and stand in a wide straddle position with your knees bent. Your legs should form a square with your knees over your ankles. If your feet are too close, then your knees will jut forward over your toes. Open the feet wider if this is the case. Make sure your knees and toes point out in the same direction. Then lift your right heel up so that you have shifted some body weight onto your right toes.

Safety Tip
If you feel any strain in your knees, open your legs farther apart.

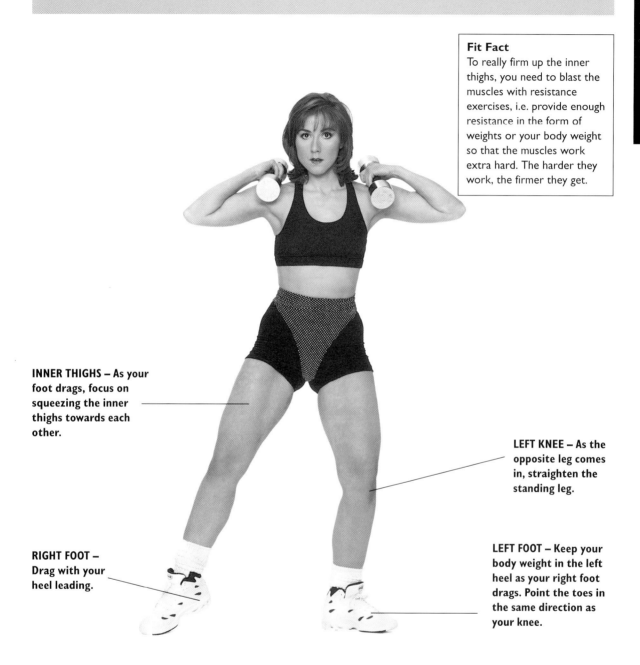

INNER THIGHS – As your foot drags, focus on squeezing the inner thighs towards each other.

LEFT KNEE – As the opposite leg comes in, straighten the standing leg.

RIGHT FOOT – Drag with your heel leading.

LEFT FOOT – Keep your body weight in the left heel as your right foot drags. Point the toes in the same direction as your knee.

Position 2. Exhale and press your right foot down into the floor and slowly drag it across towards your other leg. The foot pushing down provides extra resistance for your inner thighs as they work to close your thighs. Straighten your legs completely as your feet come together. Then inhale and reach out with the right leg and lower your hips into a wide squat. Check that your legs form a square, knees over ankles (not toes). Now press down into the floor with your left foot, drag it across and bring your thighs together.

Modification.
If you feel strain in your knee as you move the outer leg inside, release the pressure of the foot into the floor.

Gluteal Twist

The Squeeze: Focus on your buttocks during the upward and downward phase of the movement; squeeze extra tight to rotate the thigh.

Muscles worked: gluteus maximus and medius, inner thigh group

Mental Image
Imagine that your upper and lower back are a table with fine china on it. Although your leg is moving, you must make sure the table does not wobble.

BACK – Hold your torso up, rather than let it sink to the floor.

HIPS – Keep your hips even and parallel so that your abdomen faces down, not sideways.

NECK – Try not to arch your neck; look down at the floor.

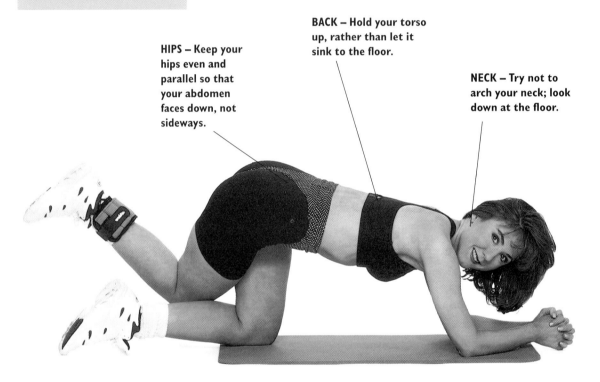

Position 1. Strap an ankle weight on or hold a light dumbbell between the calf and back of your knee. Support your body weight on your elbows and knees. Extend your right leg behind you. Cross your right knee over your left calf.

Safety Tip
Avoid lifting your leg so high that your lower back dips down and arches. Keep the movement slow and controlled.

Fit Fact
Most movements of the
upper leg are not initiated
by thigh muscles, but by
muscles in the buttocks.

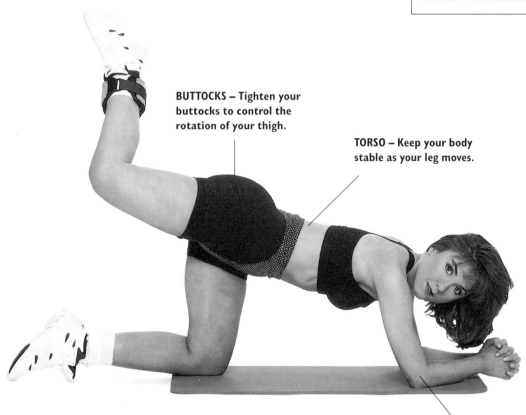

**BUTTOCKS – Tighten your
buttocks to control the
rotation of your thigh.**

**TORSO – Keep your body
stable as your leg moves.**

**ELBOWS – Distribute the
weight of your torso evenly
between your two elbows
and supporting knee.**

Position 2. As you exhale, squeeze your buttocks and lift your right leg. As it reaches hip level, rotate it outwards so that the outer thigh faces the ceiling. Lower slowly while inhaling, again crossing over the bottom calf. Repeat, then switch legs.

Modification
If you feel pain in your supporting knee, use a more padded mat or cushion or try lying across a chair or bench so that your legs can lower and lift off the edge.

75

Chapter 10

The Squeeze Exercises –
Upper Body

Arms, Back, Chest, Abdominals

Shoulder Raise

The Squeeze: Before you move tighten your shoulders to lift your arms; keep your hands light.

Muscles worked: deltoids, trapezius

Mental Image
As your arms lift, imagine that your arms are floating up. As you lower, imagine that you are pushing your arms through thick mud. Avoid dropping your arms too fast.

RIBS – Hold your ribs high off your pelvis.

ELBOWS – Keep your elbows soft.

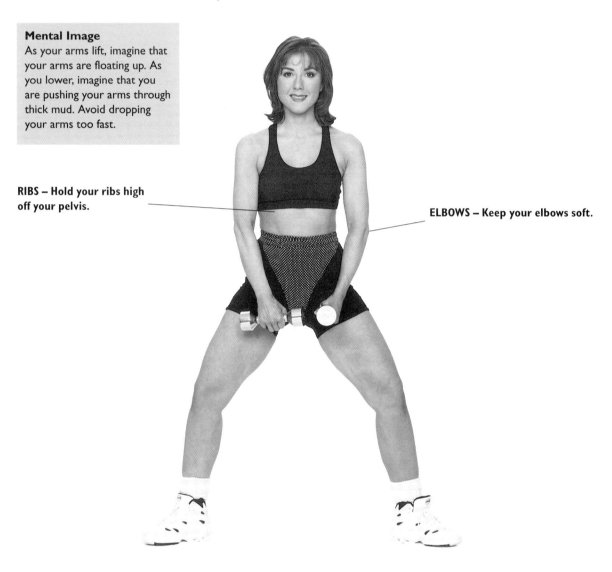

Position 1. Stand with your feet shoulder width apart, knees slightly bent. Hold the weights in front of your body, the left palm facing inwards, the right facing your thigh.

Safety Tip
Avoid arching your back or shifting your torso to hoist the weight up. If you cannot use only your arms, use a lighter weight.

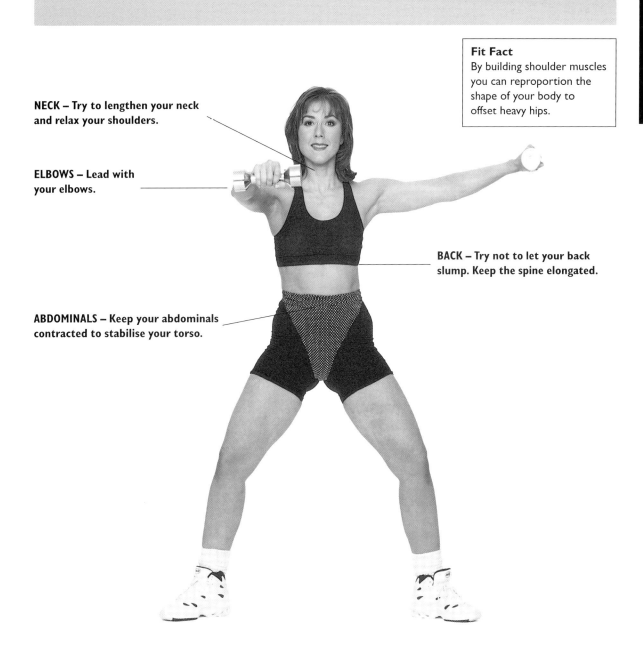

Fit Fact
By building shoulder muscles you can reproportion the shape of your body to offset heavy hips.

NECK – Try to lengthen your neck and relax your shoulders.

ELBOWS – Lead with your elbows.

BACK – Try not to let your back slump. Keep the spine elongated.

ABDOMINALS – Keep your abdominals contracted to stabilise your torso.

Position 2. As you exhale, open your left arm out to the side and lift your right arm straight out in front of you. Both hands stop when they reach shoulder level. Inhale and slowly lower your arms down in front of your thighs. As you exhale, slowly lift your hands straight out in front of you, this time alternating the direction of each, and again stopping when you reach shoulder height. Inhale, slowly lower, and repeat the sequence.

Modification.
If you find this move difficult, break it up into two separate exercises. First hold a weight in each hand and open both arms to the side. Then hold lighter weights or do fewer repetitions when you lift both arms up in front.

Biceps Curl

The Squeeze: Focus on the upper inner arm and contract the muscles as if you were pushing a button to move your hand up and down.

Muscles worked: biceps, forearms and wrist extensors

Mental Image
Picture your lower arms as two synchronised windscreen wipers on a car.

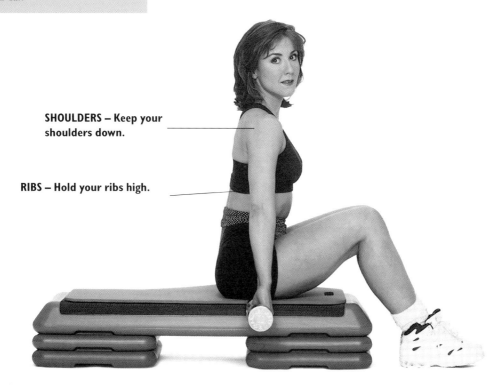

SHOULDERS – Keep your shoulders down.

RIBS – Hold your ribs high.

Position I. Sit on a bench and hold a weight in each hand. Let your arms hang by your sides with your palms facing behind you.

Safety Tip
Make sure to straighten your elbows completely, but avoid locking them.

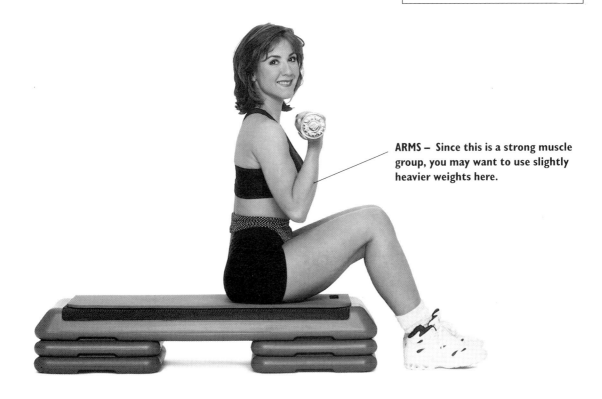

ARMS – Since this is a strong muscle group, you may want to use slightly heavier weights here.

Position 2. As you exhale, in one fluid motion bend your elbows and lift the weights to your shoulders. Turn your hands out so your palms face your chest. Inhale and rotate the palms inward as you lower.

Modification
Rather than start with your hands facing in and rotating them out, start with them turned out facing forwards. As you bend the elbow, imagine the back of your hand is sliding across an imaginary wall you are leaning against. This keeps the palm forward and stops it from rotating to face up. Lower with your palm still facing forward.

Triceps Press

The Squeeze: When the triceps shorten, the arm straightens. When they lengthen, it bends. Squeeze to control this marionette-like action.

Muscles worked: triceps, some pectoralis major, deltoids

Mental Image
Pretend that you are lying with your hands trapped under a heavy rock. As you exhale, push hard with your hands to try to lift the rock up.

ELBOWS – Try to bend your elbows as much as possible to work through a full range of motion.

ABDOMEN – Hold your abdomen in to stabilise the lower back.

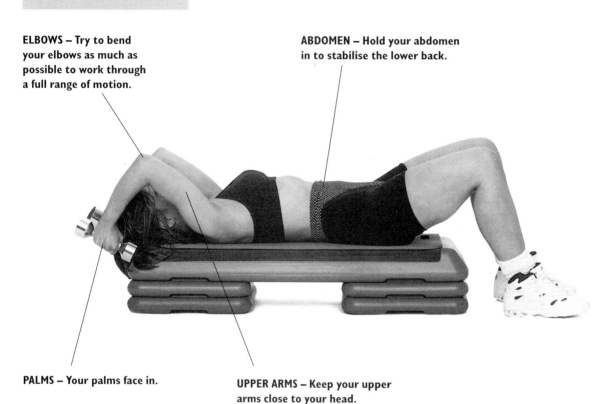

PALMS – Your palms face in.

UPPER ARMS – Keep your upper arms close to your head.

Position I. Lie on your back on a step with your knees bent, feet flat. Hold your weights above your head, then bend your elbows so that your hands drop behind your shoulders. Point your elbows slightly back rather than straight up to the ceiling.

Safety Tip
Perform this move slowly to maintain muscle control.

82

WRISTS – Keep your wrists straight, in line with your lower arm, rather than bent backward.

UPPER ARMS – Your upper arms remain still throughout; the only movement is your lower arm bending from the elbow.

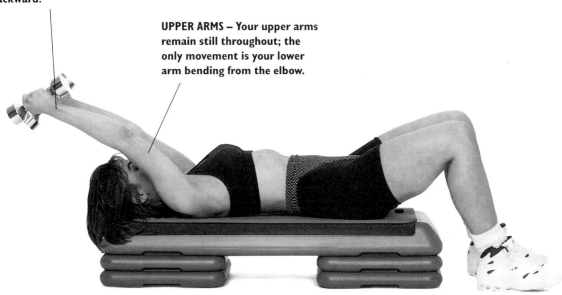

Position 2. Exhale and extend your arms until your elbows are completely straight and rotate your hands so that your palms face the ceiling. Inhale and bend your elbows again.

Modification
If you find it difficult to straighten your arms completely, use a lighter weight.

Wrist Curl

The Squeeze: Focus on the front of your lower arms. Squeeze here in order to bring the palms forward.

Muscles worked: forearm flexors

Mental Image
Pretend you are in water and trying to create a current to move towards you using only your wrists. Move your hands back and forth in a wave-like motion up and down.

Fit Fact
Strengthening the forearm and wrist can help guard against an overstress injury called repetitive stress injury which can occur from any activity in which you perform repetitive hand movements.

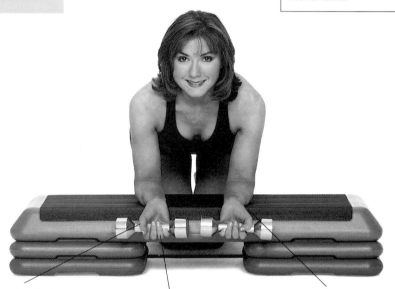

THUMBS – Keep your thumbs loose.

FINGERS – Keep a loose grip on the weight so the weights roll slightly in your hands.

FOREARMS – Keep your arms rested during the wrist action.

Position 1. Sit behind a step and rest your elbows over the edge in front of you so that your hands can hang over. Hold light weights in your hands, wrists open, palms forward.

Position 2. Exhale and lift the weights and move them towards your body by bending your wrists and turning your palms in. Inhale as you lower the weights.

Modification
Reverse this exercise by starting with your palms facing down while hanging over the edge and then bringing them up so that they face forwards to work the wrist extensors.

The Squeeze: The forearm is acting as a lever to rotate the shoulder joint. Squeeze the muscles in the shoulder throughout the movement.

Muscles worked: rotator cuff *(internal and external rotators)*

Mental Image
Imagine that your forearms are brushing across a table top as they move back and forth.

Fit Fact
After the knee, the shoulder joint is the weakest joint in the body. Therefore it is crucial to strengthen all the muscles in, on and around it.

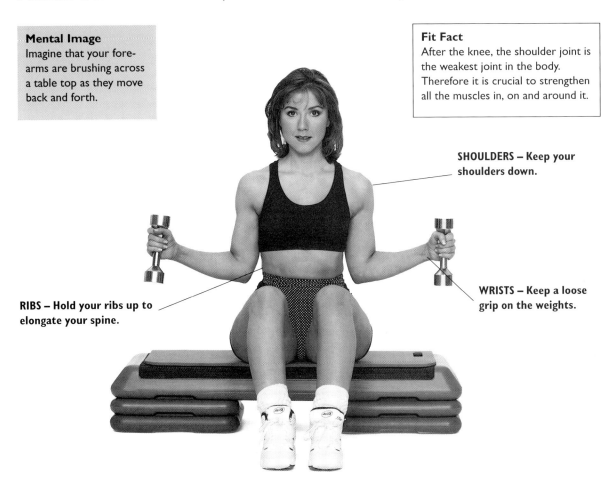

SHOULDERS – Keep your shoulders down.

WRISTS – Keep a loose grip on the weights.

RIBS – Hold your ribs up to elongate your spine.

Position 1. Sit or stand and hold light weights in your hands. Bring your elbows in to your sides and hold them close to your ribs. Your forearms should be turned out so that the back of your hands are in line with your torso, as if you were leaning against a wall.

Position 2. As you inhale, move your forearms across the front of your body until they meet. Then exhale and open your arms to the sides again. Keep your elbows close to the ribs.

Modification
These are smaller, weaker muscles, so make sure to work with a light weight or none at all.

Safety Tip
If you feel any strain in the shoulder joint, decrease the weight during this exercise.

Upper Arm Sculptor *** Advanced Exercise

The Squeeze: Concentrate on the upper arms and also be aware of the different rotations your wrists move through.

Muscles worked: biceps, triceps

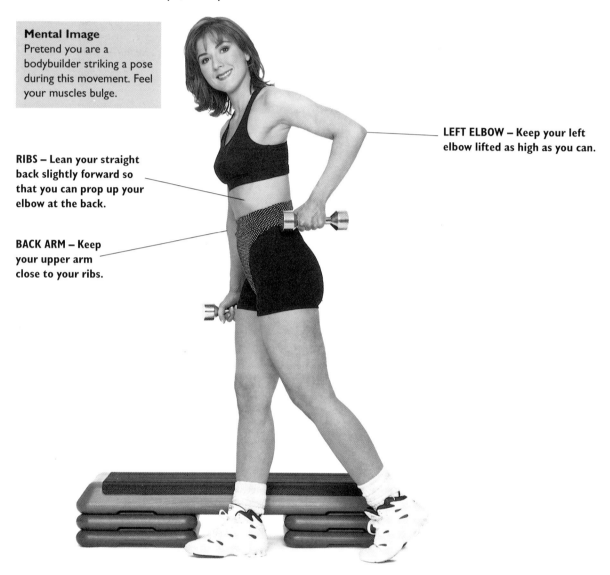

Mental Image
Pretend you are a bodybuilder striking a pose during this movement. Feel your muscles bulge.

RIBS – Lean your straight back slightly forward so that you can prop up your elbow at the back.

BACK ARM – Keep your upper arm close to your ribs.

LEFT ELBOW – Keep your left elbow lifted as high as you can.

Position 1. Stand with a weight in each hand. To start, straighten your right arm and drop it by your right thigh with your palm facing in to your thigh. At the same time, bend your left elbow and push it up behind you with the left palm facing in.

Safety Tip
Since there are several actions in opposing directions during this exercise, move more slowly than usual for better control.

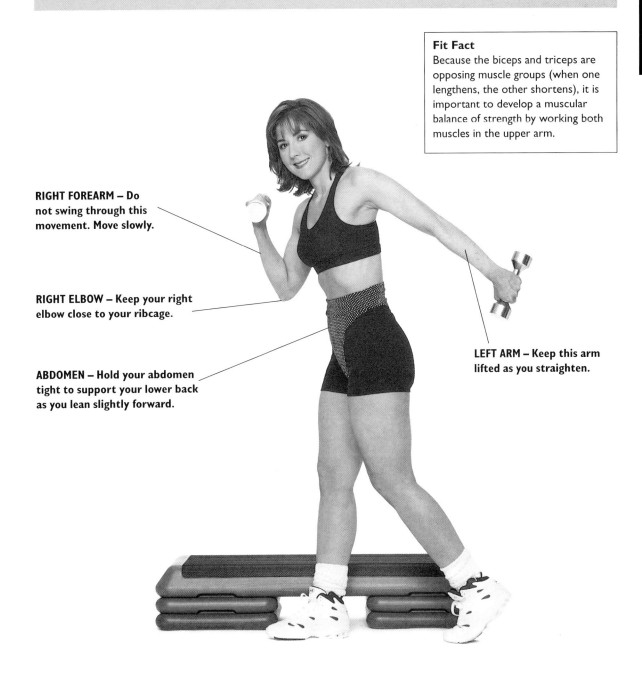

Fit Fact
Because the biceps and triceps are opposing muscle groups (when one lengthens, the other shortens), it is important to develop a muscular balance of strength by working both muscles in the upper arm.

RIGHT FOREARM – Do not swing through this movement. Move slowly.

RIGHT ELBOW – Keep your right elbow close to your ribcage.

ABDOMEN – Hold your abdomen tight to support your lower back as you lean slightly forward.

LEFT ARM – Keep this arm lifted as you straighten.

Position 2. As you exhale, bend your right elbow. Bring your right hand to your right shoulder, rotating your palm so it faces your shoulder. At the same time, straighten your left elbow at the back. Inhale and return to the starting position. Repeat, then switch sides.

Modification
Since the triceps are often weaker than the biceps, you may find this exercise easier if you use a lighter weight on your back arm.

Shoulder Row

The Squeeze: *Keep your focus on your shoulders. Squeeze these muscles extra tight to control the lowering phase.*

Muscles worked: deltoids, some trapezius, biceps

Mental Image
Pretend you have a rubber band joining your hands. As your arms move you can feel it stretching farther and farther apart. Do not let it snap back as you lower, but control the return phase of this move.

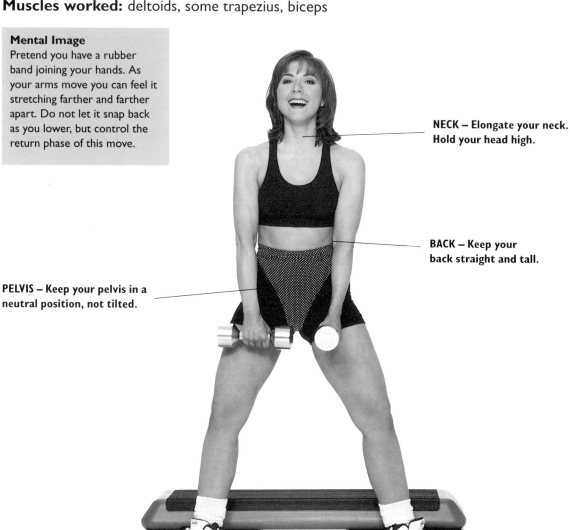

NECK – Elongate your neck. Hold your head high.

BACK – Keep your back straight and tall.

PELVIS – Keep your pelvis in a neutral position, not tilted.

Position I. Stand with your feet shoulder width apart, knees slightly bent. Hold a pair of weights in front of your legs with your right palm facing the front of your thigh and your left palm sideways, facing your right hand.

Safety Tip
Avoid scrunching your shoulders near your ears. Keep shoulders relaxed.

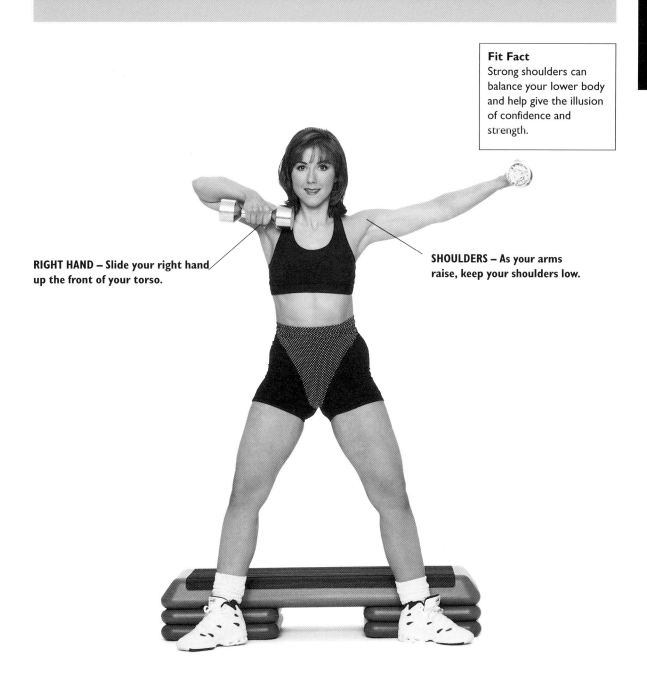

Fit Fact
Strong shoulders can balance your lower body and help give the illusion of confidence and strength.

RIGHT HAND – Slide your right hand up the front of your torso.

SHOULDERS – As your arms raise, keep your shoulders low.

Position 2. As you exhale, raise your left arm out to the side. Stop when your hand reaches shoulder level. At the same time, lift your right hand up along your chest until your elbow points to the ceiling. Inhale and slowly lower your arms in front of your thighs. Repeat, then switch sides.

Modification
You can also break this move up into two different exercises by lifting the arms in front to form a V shape as the elbows point up, or open both extended arms out to the side.

One Arm Row

The Squeeze: In the starting position, feel your back stretch. Pull with your back muscles, not your arms to raise the elbow.

Muscles worked: latissimus dorsi, rhomboids

Mental Image
Imagine that you are trying to pull the handle of a manual lawn mower. Pull slowly but with force.

Fit Fact
The most effective way to target a flabby middle is to do calorie-burning exercises such as walking or cycling to decrease the body fat. In addition you can firm up the muscles in the front and back of the waist. This exercise tones the muscles across the lower and middle back.

RIGHT ELBOW – Point your elbow up to the ceiling.

RIBS – Your ribs may rotate slightly to the right as you raise your arm.

LEFT HAND – Hold the weights loosely.

Position 1. Stand with your left leg in front of your right on a bench or the floor. Keep your front knee slightly bent. Lean on your front leg with your left arm to support your back. Hold a weight in your right hand. Allow the right arm to hang low to the floor, your palm facing your body.

Position 2. As you exhale, bend your elbow and pull the weight up to your ribcage. Keep the elbow close in to your waist as you lift. Feel your shoulder blades coming together as your elbow points up. Inhale as you slowly lower and repeat. Then switch sides.

Safety Tip
Push your forearm into your right thigh so that you are supporting the weight of your torso by leaning on your leg, not merely bending forward.

Posture Press

The Squeeze: Feel the shoulder blades lift and lower and concentrate on squeezing the shoulders and upper back.

Muscles worked: trapezius, deltoids

Mental Image
Imagine that the ceiling is as low as your head. Try to push it higher.

Fit Fact
This exercise is strenuous because it is difficult to hold weight above our heads for extended periods.

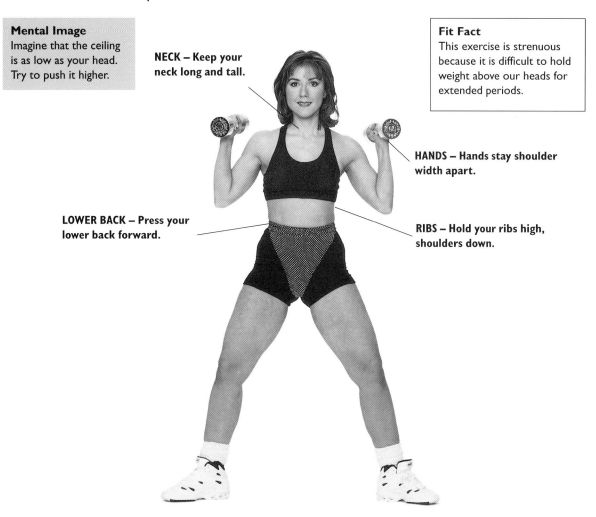

NECK – Keep your neck long and tall.

HANDS – Hands stay shoulder width apart.

LOWER BACK – Press your lower back forward.

RIBS – Hold your ribs high, shoulders down.

Position 1. Sit or stand with a weight in your hands. Hold your elbows out by your sides so that your lower arms are perpendicular to the floor. Palms face in. Lean your body slightly forward.

Position 2. Exhale and push your hands overhead to straighten your elbows. As you push up, rotate your arms until your palms face forward. Then inhale and lower your arms and turn your hands in so that they face each other. Repeat.

Modification
If your torso shifts back and forth as you raise the weight, decrease the weight.

Safety Tip
Make sure you do not arch your back by sticking your chest out as you lift your arms.

Lower Back Lift

The Squeeze: Focus on the lower back tightening as you lift.

Muscles worked: erector spinae group, gluteus maximus

Mental Image
Pretend that your back and legs
are as stiff as a piece of wood.

**FEET – Grip your feet around the
sides of the bench (or have someone else hold your feet stable).**

**BACK – Keep your back
straight, not rounded.**

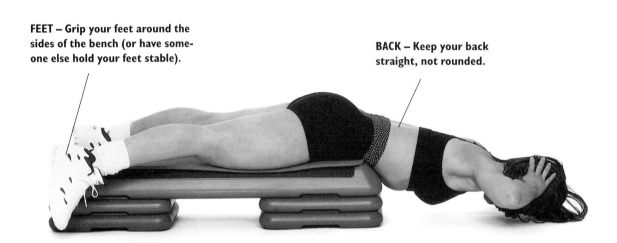

Position 1. Lie on a bench face down with your chest and waist hanging off the edge. Drop your head to the floor.

Safety Tip
Since you are working your lower back, it is natural to feel a little fatigued in the muscles. But if your back hurts, avoid lifting higher than horizontal.

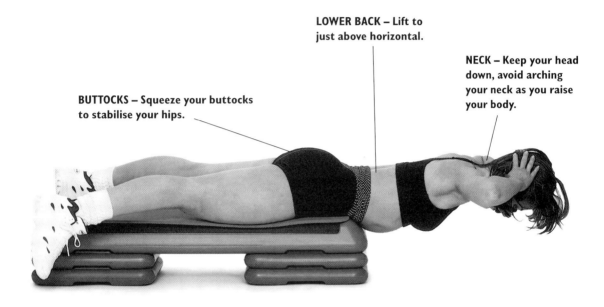

**LOWER BACK – Lift to
just above horizontal.**

**NECK – Keep your head
down, avoid arching
your neck as you raise
your body.**

**BUTTOCKS – Squeeze your buttocks
to stabilise your hips.**

Position 2. Bring your hands behind your head. As you exhale, contract the muscles in your back and buttocks to lift your chest slowly to horizontal. Lower very slowly as you inhale and repeat.

Modification
If this exercise is difficult, place your hands on your buttocks. If you feel unbalanced, do this exercise while lying flat on the floor and just lift 2 inches (5 cm) above horizontal.

Overhead Reach   ***Advanced Exercise

The Squeeze: Focus on your shoulder blade retracting as your elbow pulls in.

Muscles worked: trapezius, latissimus dorsi, rhomboids

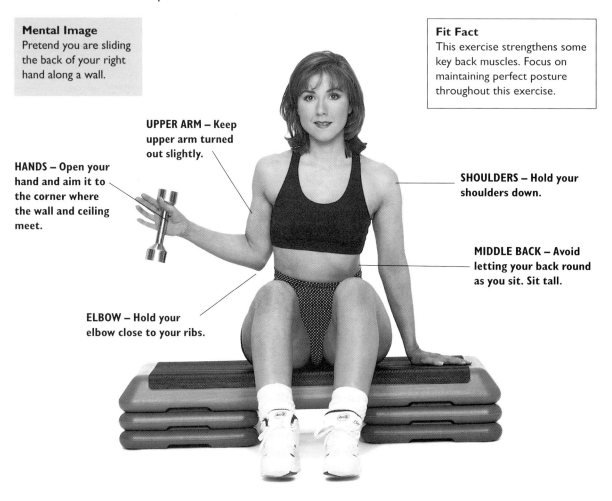

Mental Image
Pretend you are sliding the back of your right hand along a wall.

Fit Fact
This exercise strengthens some key back muscles. Focus on maintaining perfect posture throughout this exercise.

UPPER ARM – Keep upper arm turned out slightly.

HANDS – Open your hand and aim it to the corner where the wall and ceiling meet.

SHOULDERS – Hold your shoulders down.

MIDDLE BACK – Avoid letting your back round as you sit. Sit tall.

ELBOW – Hold your elbow close to your ribs.

Position 1. Sit tall and hold a light weight in your right hand on your shoulder, palm facing forward.

Position 2. As you exhale, push your hand out and up sideways so it reaches to the right corner. Then inhale and pull your elbow (not your hand) into your ribcage. Keep your hand out to the side. Repeat, then switch arms.

Modification
If you feel any strain in your shoulder joint from rotating your shoulder out, push your hand directly above your head rather than out to the side.

Safety Tip
Use a light weight if you feel strain in your shoulder.

The Squeeze: Focus on the muscles in your back and shoulders contracting through each phase. Move slowly and with control.

Muscles worked: latissimus dorsi, pectoralis major

Mental Image
Pretend that you are moving your hands through water; let them flow slowly and gracefully.

Fit Fact
Most reaching movements you make – sweeping or lifting bags – use the latissimus dorsi. It is good to work it at different angles to target more muscle fibres.

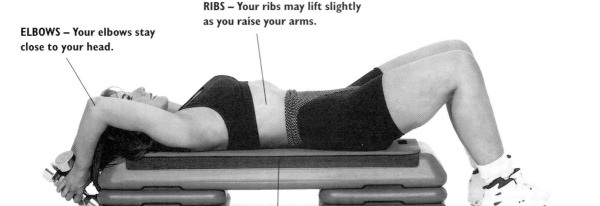

RIBS – Your ribs may lift slightly as you raise your arms.

ELBOWS – Your elbows stay close to your head.

LOWER BACK – Hold your abdomen tight to stabilise your lower back.

Position 1. Lie on your back, knees bent, feet flat. Hold a weight with both hands on top of your abdomen, elbows bent by your sides.

Position 2. Keeping your elbows close to your body, exhale and raise your hands in an arc until your hands drop behind your head. Drop your hands to the lowest comfortable point, then inhale and return to the starting position.

Modification
If your back feels strained, try not to lift your ribs during the movement.

Safety Tip
Move very slowly as you bring your arms forward and back.

95

Seated Row

The Squeeze: Feel the space in between your shoulder blades compressing so that the edges of each blade move closer together.

Muscles worked: rhomboids, posterior deltoid

Mental Image
Pretend there are strings attached to your elbows and someone standing behind you is pulling them up.

BACK – Instead of rounding your back to lean forward, concentrate on pressing the lower back to the front.

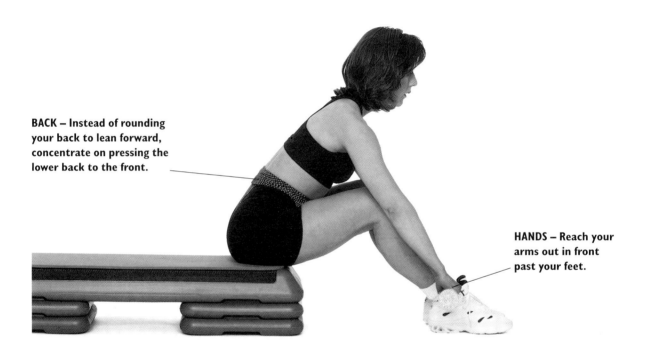

HANDS – Reach your arms out in front past your feet.

Position 1. Sit on a low bench or if you only have a chair prop your feet up so that your knees are high enough to rest on as you lean forward. Rest your chest on your thighs and hold a weight in each hand by your feet, palms facing back.

Safety Tip
If your back feels strained, tighten your abdominals and bring your feet closer to your body so that your knees provide more support to the chest.

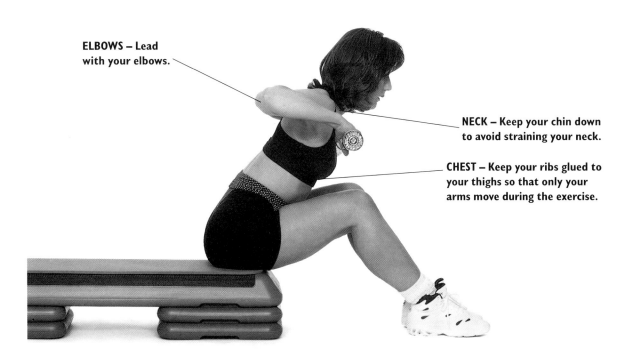

ELBOWS – Lead with your elbows.

NECK – Keep your chin down to avoid straining your neck.

CHEST – Keep your ribs glued to your thighs so that only your arms move during the exercise.

Position 2. Exhale and pull your elbows up to the ceiling. Inhale as you lower your arms.

Modification
If this feels uncomfortable, use a lighter weight or bend your elbows a little when you lift.

Safety Tip
Avoid lifting and lowering your upper torso. Keep the movement only in the arms. Remember to lean forward onto your legs so you work the back of the shoulders and upper middle back.

Back Strengthener ***Advanced Exercise

The Squeeze: Move very slowly and precisely in and out of position to feel the back muscles and buttocks articulate to produce the movement.

Muscles worked: erector spinae group, deltoids, gluteals

Mental Image
As you extend your arm and leg, try to form a perfect diagonal line. Focus on balancing as if you were a statue.

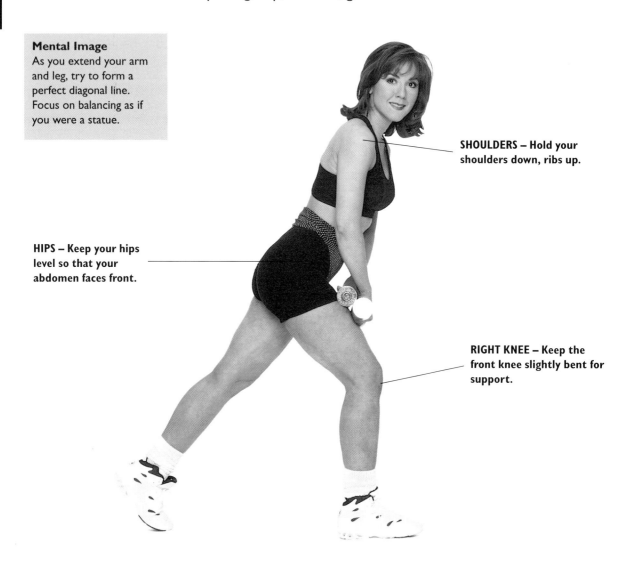

SHOULDERS – Hold your shoulders down, ribs up.

HIPS – Keep your hips level so that your abdomen faces front.

RIGHT KNEE – Keep the front knee slightly bent for support.

Position 1. Stand with your right leg slightly in front of you. Lean your straight back at a slight forward angle. Hold your weights in front of your legs. Extend your left leg behind you.

Safety Tip
You will feel the lower back muscles fatigue. Stop if you feel pain. Use a light, not heavy weight here.

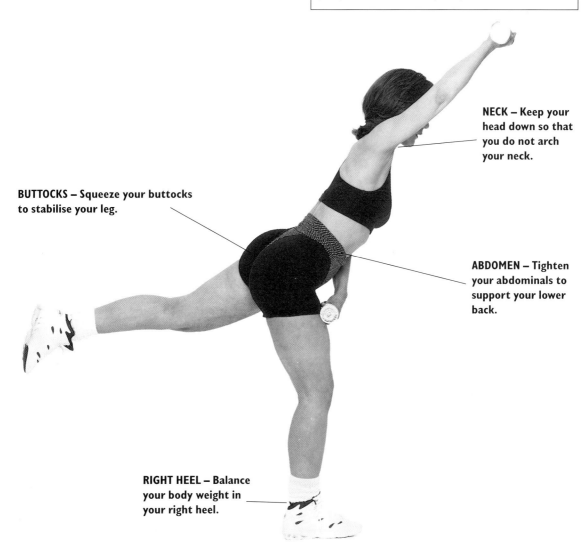

NECK – Keep your head down so that you do not arch your neck.

BUTTOCKS – Squeeze your buttocks to stabilise your leg.

ABDOMEN – Tighten your abdominals to support your lower back.

RIGHT HEEL – Balance your body weight in your right heel.

Position 2. Exhale and raise your left leg behind you as you raise your right arm in front. Hold your torso steady, chin down. You can feel muscles in the lower back contracting as you slightly arch it. Hold the extended position for a few seconds, then inhale and slowly lower your arm and leg. Then switch sides.

Modification
You may also do this exercise while lying face down on the floor. Lift the opposing arm and leg 2 inches (5 cm) off the ground.

Chest Press

The Squeeze: Drop your elbows low. Feel the pull in your pectorals, focus in and contract them. Squeeze first, then move the arms.

Muscles worked: pectorals, anterior deltoid, triceps

Mental Image
Pretend something heavy has fallen on top of you and you are trying to push it off.

HANDS – Do not squeeze the weights, but hold them lightly.

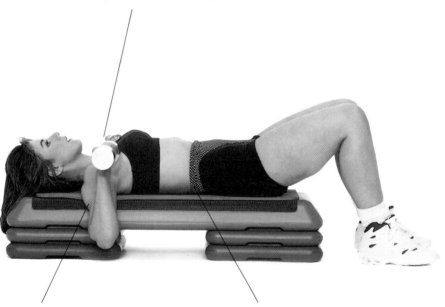

UPPER INNER ARMS – Drop your elbows low enough to stretch the muscles before each lift.

LOWER BACK – Avoid arching your back as you drop your arms.

Position 1. Lie on your back on a step or bench, knees bent. (Alternatively you can use a sofa or bed and work one arm at a time while you balance yourself with the other.) Hold the weights in your hands, palms facing your ears, elbows bent low at the sides. Hang your arms lower than the side of your step or bench so that you feel a slight stretch in your pectorals.

Safety Tip
Avoid flexing your wrists back. Hold them straight so your palms face forward. Straighten your arms, but do not lock your elbows.

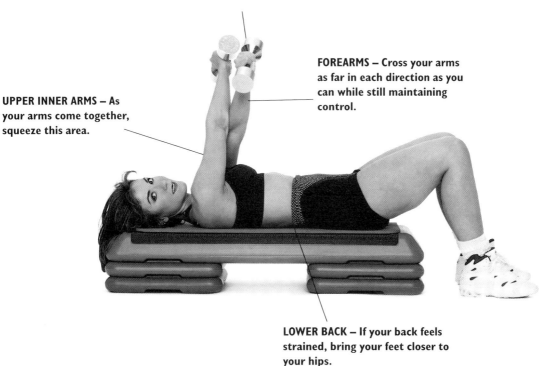

**HANDS – Avoid swinging.
Move with control.**

**FOREARMS – Cross your arms
as far in each direction as you
can while still maintaining
control.**

**UPPER INNER ARMS – As
your arms come together,
squeeze this area.**

**LOWER BACK – If your back feels
strained, bring your feet closer to
your hips.**

Position 2. As you exhale, push your hands up to the ceiling. At the highest point of the lift, cross your arms so that your elbows intersect. Hold this position for one second before you inhale and slowly lower your arms. Then repeat, alternating which arm crosses over at the top.

Modification
To make the exercise more challenging, when you cross your elbows, hold for two seconds, then lower even more slowly. If you vary the angle of your body by working on a declined or inclined step you can work more of the muscle.

Chest Squeeze

The Squeeze: Feel your elbows dropping low. As you feel them, pull in your chest muscles, focus in and contract them. Squeeze first, then move the arms together.

Muscles worked: pectorals, serratus, anterior deltoid

Mental Image
Pretend you are wrapping your arms around a giant beach ball. Try to pop it by squeezing your arms tighter.

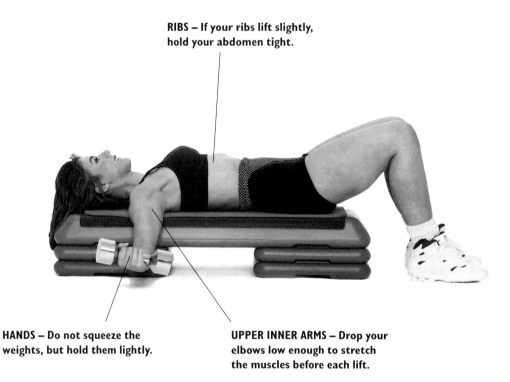

RIBS – If your ribs lift slightly, hold your abdomen tight.

HANDS – Do not squeeze the weights, but hold them lightly.

UPPER INNER ARMS – Drop your elbows low enough to stretch the muscles before each lift.

Position 1. Lie on your back on a step or bench, knees bent. Hold weights in your hands and open your arms to the sides, palms facing up. Hang your elbows lower than the side of your step.

Safety Tip
Bend your elbows more if you feel any strain in your shoulders or arms. Avoid flexing your wrists back. Hold them straight.

Fit Fact
Working all the muscles of the upper body can improve your posture, giving the illusion of bigger, perkier breasts.

HANDS – Lead with the hands on the way up, lead with the elbows on the way down.

ELBOWS – Keep your elbows slightly bent.

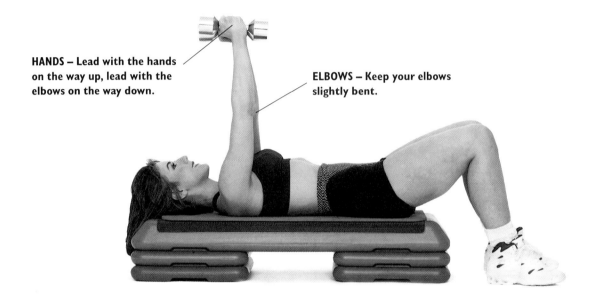

Position 2. As you exhale, move your arms in an arc until they meet over your chest. Hold for one second, then inhale and lower slowly.

Modification
Alternate the placement of your hands – over your head, chest and belly button – to work more muscle fibres.

Posture Push-Up ***Advanced Exercise

The Squeeze: Focus on your upper inner arms and on the force of your hands pushing onto the floor in order to lift.

Muscles worked: pectorals, triceps

Mental Image
Imagine that your body is a rigid board. You are trying to lift and lower it without letting it bend in the middle.

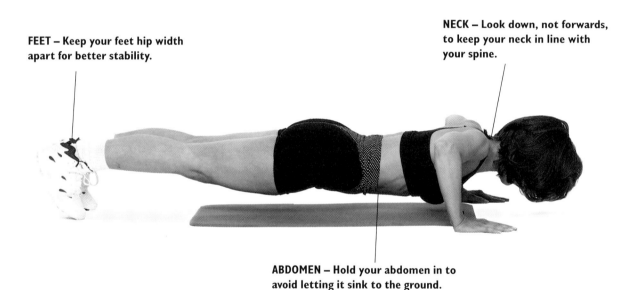

FEET – Keep your feet hip width apart for better stability.

NECK – Look down, not forwards, to keep your neck in line with your spine.

ABDOMEN – Hold your abdomen in to avoid letting it sink to the ground.

Position 1. Lie on your stomach with your hands flat on the floor just underneath your shoulders. Flex your feet so your toes push into the floor. Exhale and push your hands into the floor so you lift your entire body up, but keep your elbows bent.

Safety Tip
If you feel a burning sensation in your ribs or abdomen, it is probably the muscle fatiguing from having to hold your torso up in this position. Rest, then try again.

Fit Fact
Push yourself to develop enough strength to do a few full body push-ups, as these will strengthen many muscles in your torso.

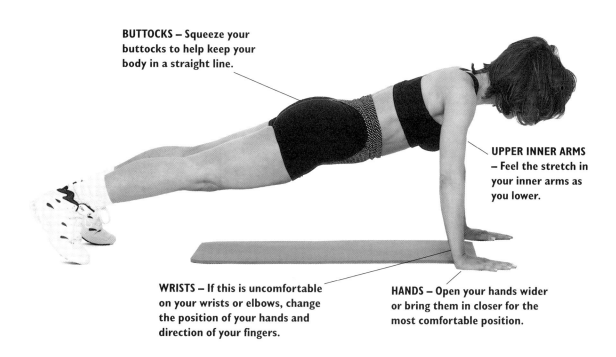

BUTTOCKS – Squeeze your buttocks to help keep your body in a straight line.

UPPER INNER ARMS – Feel the stretch in your inner arms as you lower.

WRISTS – If this is uncomfortable on your wrists or elbows, change the position of your hands and direction of your fingers.

HANDS – Open your hands wider or bring them in closer for the most comfortable position.

Position 2. As you exhale, straighten your elbows to lift your body up. Keep your hips, abdomen and ribs in a straight line. Try not to let your body sag. Inhale as you lower to the starting position (still lifted off the ground).

Modification
Try opening your feet wider or bringing them in closer for a more comfortable lift. Alternatively, you may do these push-ups while balancing on your knees instead of your toes. But this makes the exercise much less effective. So start on your knees to develop a base level of strength. Then progress by doing one full body push-up perfectly. Add one more each week as you become stronger.

Crunch

The Squeeze: Concentrate on the muscle which runs from your ribs to pubic bone. Tighten it to pull the lower ribs towards your hip bones.

Muscles worked: rectus abdominus, possibly transversus abdominus

Mental Image
Imagine your rectus abdominus contracting like an accordion as you compress your ribcage and pelvic girdle. When you reach the top of the lift, pretend there is a lid on top of your torso. Press it tightly on top of your body when you flatten your abdomen.

Fit Fact
Flattening your abdomen makes an exercise more difficult. Some experts attribute this to another abdominal muscle which may be activated, the transverse abdominus. Since it is the deepest abdominal muscle, no studies have been able to measure it. But it is likely that when it compresses it provides extra resistance making the exercise more challenging.

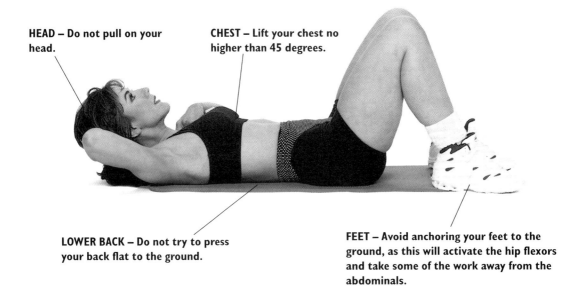

HEAD – Do not pull on your head.

CHEST – Lift your chest no higher than 45 degrees.

LOWER BACK – Do not try to press your back flat to the ground.

FEET – Avoid anchoring your feet to the ground, as this will activate the hip flexors and take some of the work away from the abdominals.

Position 1. Lie on your back with your knees bent. Bring one hand behind your head and lift your shoulder blades 2 inches (5 cm) off the ground. Hold a weight just below your neck with the other hand. Keep your chin away from your chest. Notice the contraction of your abdominal muscles in this position.

Position 2. As you exhale, flatten your abdominals, then bring your ribcage towards your hips. Keep your chin open. At the highest point, intensify the squeeze by focusing on the muscles in your abdomen and flattening them without lifting any higher. Inhale and slowly lower so that your shoulder blades touch down but your head stays lifted slightly up. Lift again.

Safety Tip
Avoid resting your head on the floor in between each lift as this may strain the neck when you lift again.

Waist Twist

The Squeeze: Focus on the deep muscles underneath each hip bone. Consciously contract the muscles before you move in order to turn to the side.

Muscles worked: internal and external obliques

Mental Image
Imagine your ribs rotating to each side. Pretend you are putting your hands in your pockets. Turn your shoulders in the direction that your fingers would slide.

Fit Fact
It is quite easy to pull too hard on your head. Try to rest your head in your palms like a pillow to support your neck through the lift.

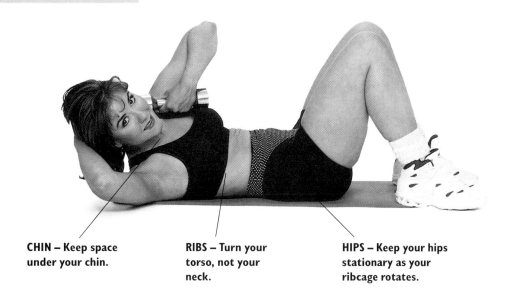

CHIN – Keep space under your chin.

RIBS – Turn your torso, not your neck.

HIPS – Keep your hips stationary as your ribcage rotates.

Position 1. Lie on your back with your legs bent, feet flat. Bring your right hand behind your head and hold a weight on your shoulder with your left hand.

Position 2. As you exhale, turn your left shoulder towards your right thigh. At the same time, tilt your right hip towards your shoulder. Your hip and opposite rib compress towards each other. Inhale and lower extra slowly. Repeat on the other side.

Modification
Eliminate the hip action and keep the pelvis stable if you feel the move is difficult to control.

Safety Tip
Avoid pulling on your head with your right hand.

Reverse Curl

The Squeeze: First consciously contract the abdominal muscles, then use them to pull your hips forward.

Muscles worked: rectus abdominus, possibly transversus abdominus

Mental Image
Imagine a big balloon resting on top of your torso. Your hips and shoulders are the only grip on the balloon. You must squeeze these areas tight to keep it from floating away.

Fit Fact
Many people think that the upper and lower abdomen are two separate muscles. In fact, there is just one long muscle which extends all the way down the torso, the rectus abdominus.

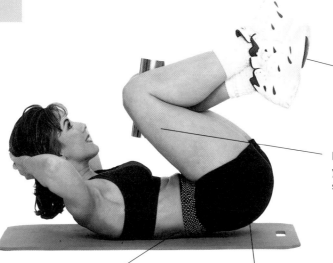

FEET – Keep the focus on the abdomen squeezing rather than the legs lifting.

LEGS – Keep legs held into your chest as if they were superglued into place.

LOWER BACK – Keep your back on the ground. Tilt only the pelvis.

TAILBONE – At first the end of your spine points away from your body. As you tilt it points up to the ceiling.

Position 1. Lie on your back and bend your knees into your chest. Bring your hands behind your head. Place a light weight in between your knees. If you feel any strain in your lower back, eliminate the weight.

Position 2. As you exhale, tighten your abdominal muscles and bring the weight closer to your chest by tilting your pelvis forward. At the same time, bring your chest closer to your hips. Hold, then flatten your abdominals to the floor for one second. Inhale and slowly release your abdominals so that your tailbone lowers to the floor.

Modification
Bring your hands flat by your sides for stability. Then move only the lower body.

Safety Tip
Avoid swinging your back off the ground. Move slowly to avoid relying on momentum to move the pelvis.

The Squeeze: Focus on the waist and squeeze the muscle fibres even as you lower.

Muscles worked: obliques

Mental Image
Imagine that you have a string attached to the side of your lower ribs which is being pulled towards your hip.

Fit Fact
Although most of the muscle fibres in the obliques run diagonally across the body, there are a few on the outer parts of the muscles which run vertically. When these contract, they shorten and bend the ribs closest to the hips. This exercise targets those fibres.

WAIST – Compress the waist area.

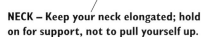

NECK – Keep your neck elongated; hold on for support, not to pull yourself up.

Position 1. Lie on your right side with your right arm along the front of your body. Bend your knees. Hold your left hand behind your head.

Position 2. Exhale and move your ribcage and hips closer together. Rather than trying to yank on your neck, concentrate on moving your ribcage closer to your top hip. This is a very subtle movement. Inhale and separate your ribs from your hips. Repeat, then switch sides.

Modification
If you find this too difficult to manoeuvre, you can also lie on your back with your knees bent, feet flat. Drop your knees to one side and lift your ribs towards the opposite side.

Safety Tip
Keep this movement very subtle and precise.

Reverse Twist ***Advanced Exercise

The Squeeze: Focus on the lower abdomen to tilt and turn the pelvis

Muscles worked: obliques, rectus abdominus

Mental Image
Imagine that your feet are walking on the ceiling. First they move towards your head. Then they turn slightly to one side. Bring them parallel again, then a little way back, then forward again and turned in the other direction.

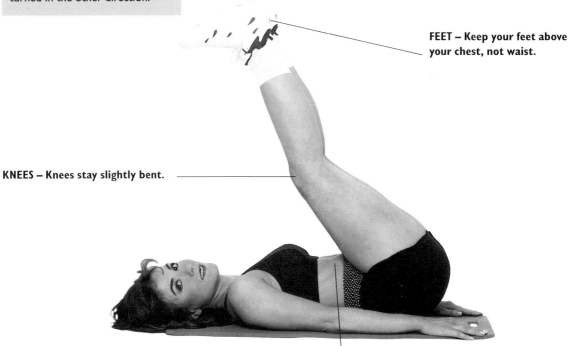

FEET – Keep your feet above your chest, not waist.

KNEES – Knees stay slightly bent.

HIPS – Contract your abdominals to stabilise your pelvis.

Position 1. Lie on your back with your arms resting on the floor. Bring your knees to your chest then straighten your legs up towards the ceiling.

Safety Tip
If you feel pain in your lower back, check to see that your knees are slightly bent and your legs are staying over your ribs. Avoid twisting so far over to each side that you lose control and put too much torque on the lower back.

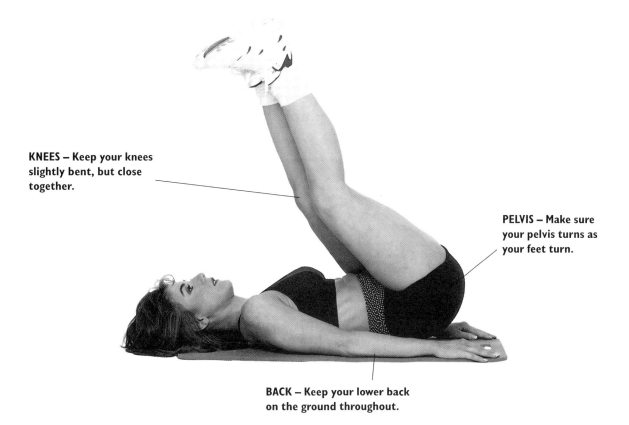

KNEES – Keep your knees slightly bent, but close together.

PELVIS – Make sure your pelvis turns as your feet turn.

BACK – Keep your lower back on the ground throughout.

Position 2. Exhale and contract your abdomen to tilt your pelvis as you would in a standard reverse curl (see page 108), but then activate your obliques by tilting your right hip towards the left side of your ribs. Inhale, then release very slowly. Then bring your left hip toward the right. The movement is very precise.

Modification
If you find this move too difficult, bend your knees.

Knee Drop ***Advanced Exercise

The Squeeze: Pause at each side and focus on the lower abdomen. Squeeze the abdominal muscles as if they were a button you push in order to move the legs.

Muscles worked: obliques, rectus abdominus

Mental Image
Imagine that you are drawing a half circle with your knees as you bring them from side to side.

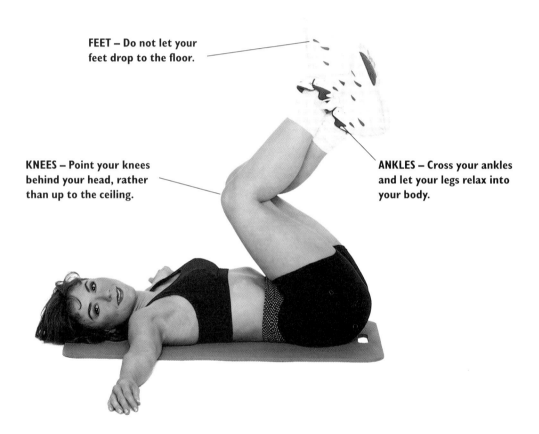

FEET – Do not let your feet drop to the floor.

KNEES – Point your knees behind your head, rather than up to the ceiling.

ANKLES – Cross your ankles and let your legs relax into your body.

Position 1. Lie on your back with your knees bent into your chest. Open your arms and place them out by your sides.

Safety Tip
This is an advanced exercise, so make sure that you are able to perform the other abdominal exercises with good form and control before you try this one.

RIBS – Keep the ribcage stable throughout this move.

BACK – If your back feels strained when you lower your legs, keep the knees high on the floor in the direction of your shoulders.

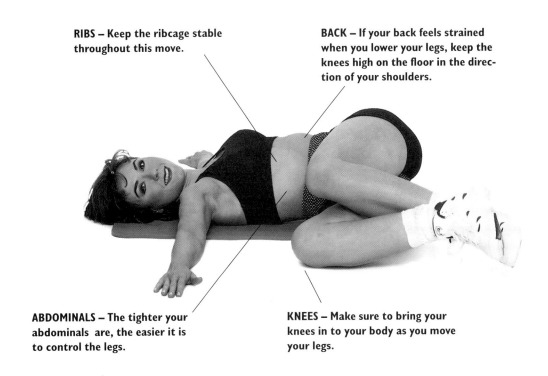

ABDOMINALS – The tighter your abdominals are, the easier it is to control the legs.

KNEES – Make sure to bring your knees in to your body as you move your legs.

Position 2. As you exhale, *slowly* lower your thighs to one side. Inhale while the legs are resting, then exhale and *slowly* contract your abdominals to lift your legs and move them back to your chest. Repeat on the other side.

Modification
If you find this move difficult to control, decrease the range of motion. Make sure that your arms are a stable base of support and tilt the legs only partly to the side rather than all the way to the floor. As you get stronger, increase the depth of the drop.

Chapter 11

The Stretches

The Stretches

Whether you are sitting, standing or running, there are always some muscles working in your body. When you move, various muscles contract, or shorten, causing your limbs to move in different directions. This muscular tension gives your body support, and also keeps your muscles firm and strong. But sometimes you can hold *too much* tension in your body. This can cause you to feel stiff and tight. If you overexercise or fail to work your muscles in a full range of motion (bend and straighten your arm only part way during a biceps curl, for example), you may gradually decrease your flexibility.

You can even develop excess tension unconsciously. If you are mentally stressed, for example, you may unconsciously hunch your shoulders up to your ears, or clench facial muscles by furrowing your brow or tightening your jaw. Muscles that stay tight can lead to postural imbalances, so it is important to have a balance in your routine. As well as tightening your muscles through strength and endurance exercise, you need to relax them by stretching.

Stretching is simply positioning your body in such a way that a particular muscle lengthens. After sleeping all night in the same position for up to ten hours, on waking your natural instinct is to stretch. When a cat has been sitting for a long period, as it rises, it will luxuriously stretch one leg, then the other, before walking away. Stretching not only feels good, but also increases your overall flexibility and suppleness. You'll feel more mobile; loose rather than tight.

When you lengthen your muscles you not only relieve muscular tension but also loosen some of the connective tissue in a joint. So stretching is a great way to release trapped tension in a muscle. You'll feel more relaxed by having a good stretch after an intense exercise session.

But it's important to realise that stretching alone is not enough to keep your body fit. Even those exercise programmes which involve a lot of stretching (yoga and ballet) have an equal amount of strengthening too. Some exercise regimes portray stretching as a cure-all and some quack 'techniques' even claim that it will help burn fat and reshape your body. This is impossible, since stretching burns very few calories and does not make your muscles firmer, only looser.

Many people believe that regular stretching will help decrease your chances of injury from exercise. While there is no research to prove this, it will help your body feel better – looser and more agile as you move.

Some people also believe that stretching can also alter your body shape by making your muscles longer. This is false too. Stretching *will* lengthen your muscle fibres, but only temporarily. Long and short muscles are hereditary; you cannot alter your genetic makeup. Generally the taller you are, the leaner you'll look.

When to Stretch

Many people enjoy doing a few stretches before and after a vigorous exercise session. Others prefer to perform stretches in more relaxed settings apart from their regular workouts. Both methods are fine. The US governing body of exercise, the American College of Sports Medicine, recommends that you stretch at least three times a week. Since you only need to spend 20 or 30 seconds on each stretch, this amounts to only 5–10 minutes a session to stretch out all the major muscles in your body.

Warm Up

Your tissues are more easily stretched when they are warm. So it is best to stretch after you have done 'warm up' exercises such as marching in place and moving your arms and legs rhythmically in different directions. Or you can save your flexibility sessions for after the workout, rather than before, when your muscles are already warm. On cold days, or in the mornings when your body temperature may be lower than normal, make sure to do a slightly longer warm up.

Warming up is not only important to stretching, but research has shown that your muscles will respond better to exercise if you prepare them first by easing them slowly into a more intense workload. By doing gentle exercise before you push yourself hard, your joints will become lubricated, you'll speed up your blood circulation and other conditions in your body will improve so that your body functions as efficiently as possible during more vigorous exercise sessions.

There is no one set way to warm up. Generally, the easiest thing to do is to start your chosen activity very slowly. If you were going to go running, say, you would walk for about five minutes. If you were going to go cycling, you would cycle very slowly for five minutes. If you were playing a sport or taking a fitness class, your warm up could be as simple as marching in place and walking while simulating some of the arm movements you'd use in the activity later on.

If in doubt about how to warm up, just march on the spot or walk slowly, while adding simple arm movements such as shoulder circles and reaching your arms in different directions for five minutes. Then follow your warm up by doing the following slow stretches.

The Stretches

These stretches target most of the key muscle groups you'll be using.

The way you stretch is important. Avoid bouncing or *forcing* your body to stretch. Instead, hold a stretch gently. Do not 'pulse'. Start with an easy rather than deep stretch.

If you feel any pain whatsoever, that's a sign that you've pushed yourself too far. Many people believe that they are so inflexible that they need to stretch harder in order to compensate. In my classes I've seen people yanking and pulling on various body parts to increase their stretch. This defeats the whole purpose. If you are having to exert force to stretch, then your muscles will respond by tightening, not relaxing.

When you begin a stretch, focus on the muscle. You'll notice after 15–20 seconds a subtle release of tension. Then, and only then, should you try to stretch a little further. If you do not feel the muscles loosen, then it may take a few sessions before you are ready to do more. Don't worry about seeing dramatic increases, for stretching is about relaxation. You may wish to use deep breathing and relaxing music during your sessions. The calmer your approach, the more flexible you will become.

But keep in mind that you can be too flexible. There is absolutely no need to become as flexible as a dancer or yoga guru. If you are able to twist your body into pretzel-like positions, you may have even overstretched your ligaments. Ligaments are different from muscles or tendons. Their function is to hold bones together for stability. Once a ligament is overstretched it may never give you adequate support around a joint. This leaves you more susceptible to injury. If you've ever sprained a knee ligament, for example, you may have permanent wobbling and permanent weakness. Stretch enough so you feel pleasurable waves of tension release, not strain.

Hold each of the following stretches for 10–30 seconds. Exhale as you stretch to help the muscle relax.

Back and Neck Tension Reliever

Mental Image
Feel the weight of your head sink down like a limb hanging from a tree.

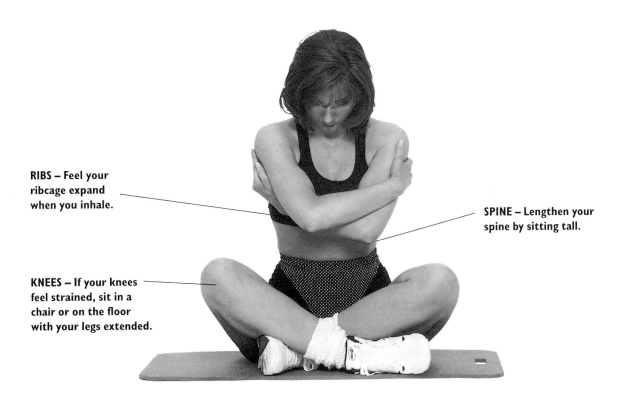

RIBS – Feel your ribcage expand when you inhale.

SPINE – Lengthen your spine by sitting tall.

KNEES – If your knees feel strained, sit in a chair or on the floor with your legs extended.

Position I. Sit cross-legged on the floor. Hold your shoulders down and hug yourself. Drop your chin slightly. Inhale so that your ribcage expands. Notice your shoulder blades moving apart and stretching the muscles in your upper back.

Position 2. Hold your shoulders down and gently allow your head to drop towards your right shoulder. Hold until you feel some of the tension release from the muscles in your neck, then carefully allow your head to roll in front to bring your left ear to your left shoulder.

Safety Tip
Do not let your lower back sink. Keep your spine erect and tall as you stretch the upper back.

Hip and Bum Stretch

Mental Image
Imagine your lower leg is a lever which you can move forward and backward to adjust the stretch.

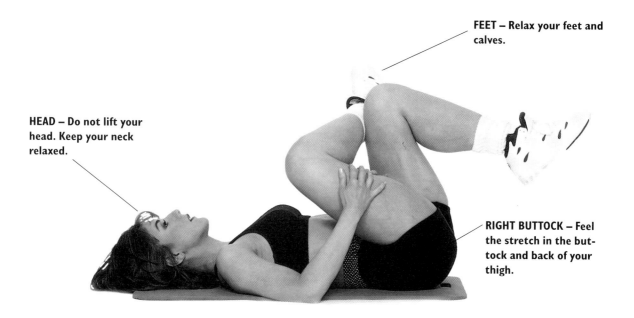

FEET – Relax your feet and calves.

HEAD – Do not lift your head. Keep your neck relaxed.

RIGHT BUTTOCK – Feel the stretch in the buttock and back of your thigh.

Position 1. Lie on your back and cross your right leg over your left. Turn your top knee slightly out to the right side. Hold your left thigh in to your chest. Hold, then switch sides.

Safety Tip
If your knee feels uncomfortable put your calf on top of the bottom knee so that your top foot points forward rather than out to the side.

Back Thigh and Calf Stretch

Mental Image
Imagine that the muscles in the back of your leg are melting and becoming longer.

BACK – Lean your back slightly forward, but do not drop your chest.

HIPS – Push your hips behind you to increase the stretch.

FRONT KNEE – Keep your front knee slightly bent.

Position 1. Stand and place your right foot on a bench or chair. Lift your ribcage and lean slightly forward. Support the weight of your torso by placing your hands on your front leg. Press your lower back toward the front thigh. When the back of your front thigh relaxes, flex your toes forwards to your shin so you feel a deeper stretch in the calf. Hold, then switch sides.

Safety Tip
Do not worry about touching your head or chest to your knees as this may cause you to round your lower back and strain it. If you feel pain in your calf, drop your toes back and bend the front knee slightly to decrease the stretch.

121

Torso Stretch

Mental Image
Imagine that your torso is a plant. Look up to the sun and feel your top arm and chest lifting towards it to soak up the light.

NECK – Turn your neck out with your chest, but if it feels strained, keep it down.

RIBS – Lift your ribs away from your hips.

SPINE – Do not try to bend over to the side; instead, lift up.

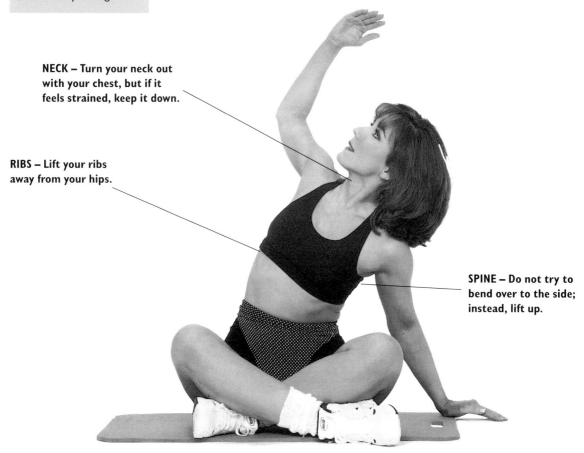

Position 1. Sit cross-legged. Lift your right arm to the ceiling and open your chest. Hold the stretch until you feel the muscles in your side relax. Switch sides.

Safety Tip
If your back feels strained, make sure you support the weight of your upper body by leaning on your bottom hand.

Mental Image
Imagine you are a
big baboon puffing
up its chest.

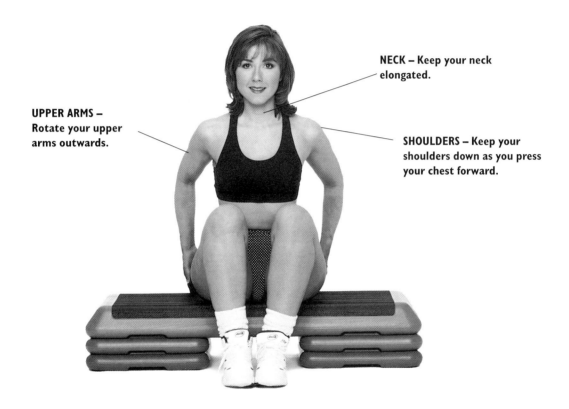

NECK – Keep your neck
elongated.

UPPER ARMS –
Rotate your upper
arms outwards.

SHOULDERS – Keep your
shoulders down as you press
your chest forward.

Position I. Sit on a bench, arms by your side. Rotate your palms out to open your arms, then bring your arms behind you. Hold your ribs up high as you sit. Press your hands against the back of the bench to resist against as you press your shoulders forward to stretch your chest muscles.s

Safety Tip
If your back feels strained, then sit or stand next to a wall. Place your hands on the wall at shoulder level, then press your chest forward.

Upper Arm and Shoulder Stretch

Mental Image
Push your elbow up to the ceiling as if there were a string attached pulling it upwards.

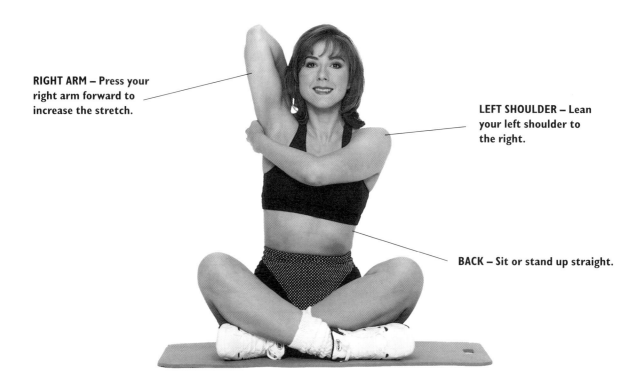

RIGHT ARM – Press your right arm forward to increase the stretch.

LEFT SHOULDER – Lean your left shoulder to the right.

BACK – Sit or stand up straight.

Position1. Straighten your right arm up to the ceiling then drop your hand behind your shoulder. Reach your left hand across your body in front, then reach around your side to hold on to the right hand. Feel the stretch in the back of your upper arm and front of your left shoulder.

Safety Tip
If you find it difficult to grasp your back hand, hold on to the shoulder instead.

Hip and Thigh Stretch

Mental Image
Exhale and imagine that your left hip is sinking in quicksand.

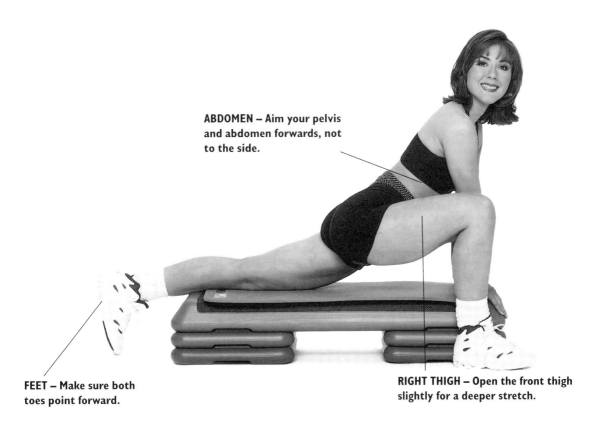

ABDOMEN – Aim your pelvis and abdomen forwards, not to the side.

FEET – Make sure both toes point forward.

RIGHT THIGH – Open the front thigh slightly for a deeper stretch.

Position 1. Stand with your feet shoulder width apart, then bring your right leg in front along the side of a step. (If you do not have a step, you can rest your leg on the floor or keep it propped up by supporting your body weight on your hands.) Bend your right knee and drop your pelvis so that your back leg rests on the bench. Press your left hip forward so you feel a stretch in the area where your pelvis and upper thigh connect. When these muscles release, lift your left foot slightly so you feel a stretch in the front of your left thigh. Hold, then switch sides.

Safety Tip
If you feel pain in your front knee, straighten your back leg more. The knee should be at a 90-degree angle over your ankle, not toes.

125

Lower Back Stretch

Mental Image
Feel your spine rotate gently and imagine that your chest is the front of a leaf turning up towards the sun.

NECK – Hold your chin down to avoid arching your neck.

INNER THIGHS – Push your hips back to feel a stretch in the inner thighs as well.

LEFT HAND – Press your body weight into your hand.

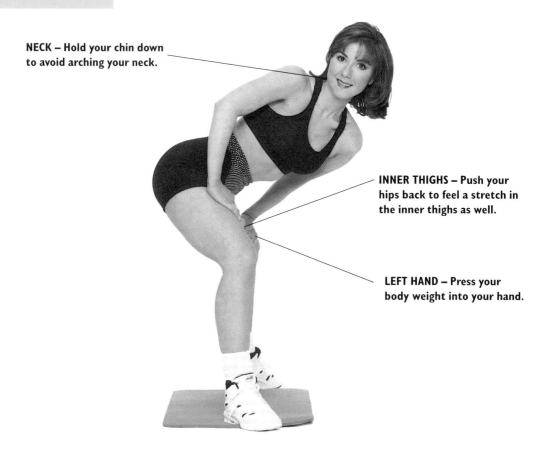

Position1. Stand in a wide straddle position with your knees slightly bent. Lean forward at an angle and support the weight of your torso by leaning your hands on your thighs. Press your left shoulder and chest forward as you look to the right. Hold, then switch sides.

Safety Tip
Keep your back straight, not rounded.

Back of the Thigh and Inner Thigh Stretch

Mental Image
Imagine that the muscles in the back and inner thigh are pieces of chewing gum which you can stretch to become longer and longer.

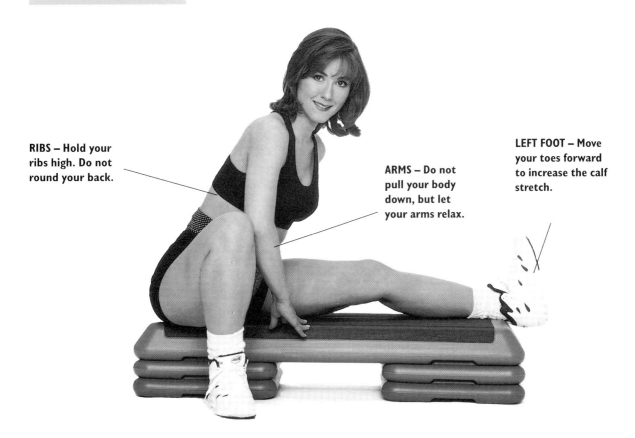

RIBS – Hold your ribs high. Do not round your back.

ARMS – Do not pull your body down, but let your arms relax.

LEFT FOOT – Move your toes forward to increase the calf stretch.

Position 1. Sit on a bench in a wide straddle position with your left leg extended on the bench and your right leg bent. Press your lower back and chest towards the straight leg. Hold the stretch as the backs of your thighs relax.

Position 2. Lift your torso up and turn your body towards the right. Lean forward to feel the stretch in your inner thigh.

Safety Tip
Do not round the back or try to touch your head to your knee.

Chapter 12

Your Personalised Squeeze Routine

Your Personalised Squeeze Routine

You can either choose a selection of *Squeeze* exercises to include in your regular routine or follow one of the programmes I have outlined below:

1. Choose your fitness level from Chart 1.
2. Choose which *Squeeze* routine to follow from Chart 2.
3. If you are following Routine B or C, then refer to page 46 to determine your starting weight.
4. Choose one to three whole body activities from Chart 3.
5. Plug your whole body activities and *Squeeze* routine into your weekly schedule (Chart 4).

CHART 1: YOUR FITNESS LEVEL

This chart will help you determine what level you are at.

Level 1: Without Weights

If you have not exercised in a year or longer, start Routine A at this level. Some exercises will be very easy for you; some will be quite difficult. This is because some muscles are naturally stronger than others. Also, some of the arm exercises will not be difficult without the added resistance of weights. During the easier exercises, focus on intensifying how hard your muscles are moving. During the harder exercises, do not worry if you can only do two or three repetitions. Gradually increase by one or two reps each week.

When you can get through these exercises comfortably, with precision and control, you are ready to progress to Routine B and try the exercises with weights.

Level 1: With Weights

If you have not exercised in six months or more, start Routine B at this level. It is recommended you go through the *Squeeze* exercises at least once without weights to perfect your form before trying them with weights. Start using weights which are 2–5 lb (1–2 kg).

When you can get through two sets of these exercises comfortably, with precision and control, aim to increase your resistance a bit more (either by adding more weight or working harder). Finally, when you can perform with strength and control, progress to Routine C.

Level 2: With Weights

If you are already familiar with weights and exercising at least two days a week, start at Routine B: With Weights to master the basic moves. When you feel confident, go through the more advanced exercises in Routine C without weights the first few times so that you can master the technique. When you can complete one set of the exercises, you may wish to intensify the workout by doing another set of each of the moves or by increasing your weight resistance.

CHART 2 : YOUR SQUEEZE ROUTINE

Routine A	*Routine B*	*Routine C*
Squat	Squat	Squat Kick
Hamstring Curl	Hamstring Curl	Inner Thigh Tightener
Leg Reach	Leg Reach	Gluteal Twist
Gluteal Twist	Gluteal Twist	Calf Raise
Calf Raise	Calf Raise	
Shoulder Raise	Shoulder Raise	Shoulder Raise
Biceps Curl	Biceps Curl	Upper Arm Sculptor
Wrist Curl	Wrist Curl	Rotator Cuff
One Arm Row	One Arm Row	One Arm Row
Posture Press	Posture Press	Posture Press
Overhead Reach	Lower Back Lift	Overhead Reach
Seated Row	Seated Row	Seated Row
Chest Squeeze	Chest Squeeze	Pullover
	Chest Press	Back Strengthener
		Chest Press
		Posture Push-Up
Crunch	Crunch	Crunch
Waist Twist	Waist Twist	Waist Twist
	Reverse Curl	Side Lift
		Reverse Twist
		Knee Drop
Estimated Time:	Estimated Time:	Estimated Time:
40–50 minutes	40–50 minutes	40–60 minutes

* See Chart 5 (page 136) to find out which page these exercises are on.

CHART 3: WHOLE BODY ACTIVITIES

The following are everyday whole body activities. Choose one to three that would be convenient and easy for you to do regularly. Then plug them into your weekly schedule.

walking	jogging	cycling	swimming
rowing	tennis	dancing	squash
golf (without a cart)	ice skating	roller skating	badminton
stair machine	fitness video	step class	aerobics class
aqua aerobics			

Your Personalised Squeeze Routine

CHART 4: YOUR WEEKLY SCHEDULE

The following schedule shows what you should do on two to four days during a seven-day week. You can choose which days of the week to slot your exercise sessions into. You may do your whole body exercises on consecutive days, but make sure that you leave a day in between your *Squeeze* sessions. So you would not do your *Squeeze* exercises on Monday and Tuesday, say, rather Monday and Wednesday. Do not do *Squeeze* sessions more than three days per week. I have included some days where you do only a whole body workout, others where you do only the *Squeeze* workout and others where you do both. If you have trouble exercising more than just a few days a week, you can combine the separate days. Remember to do a warm up and do *Squeeze* stretches at least twice a week (see Chapter 11) or you can do them before and after each session.

Routine A

Week	Day 1	Day 2	Day 3	Day 4
1	whole body 10 mins	*Squeeze* 1 set, 10 reps	*Squeeze* 1 set, 10 reps; whole body 10 mins	rest
2	whole body 10"	*Squeeze* 1 set, 12 reps	*Squeeze* 1 set, 12 reps; whole body 12"	rest
3	whole body 12"	*Squeeze* 1 set, 12 reps	*Squeeze* 1 set, 12 reps; whole body 15"	rest
4	whole body 15"	*Squeeze* 1 set, 15 reps	*Squeeze* 1 set, 15 reps; whole body 15"	rest
5	*Squeeze* 2 sets, 10 reps	whole body 15"	rest	*Squeeze* 2 sets, 10 reps; whole body 15"
6	*Squeeze* 2 sets, 10 reps	whole body 18"	rest	*Squeeze* 2 sets, 10 reps; whole body 18"
7	*Squeeze* 2 sets, 12 reps	whole body 18"	rest	*Squeeze* 2 sets, 12 reps; whole body 18"

8	*Squeeze* 2 sets, 12 reps	whole body 20"	rest	*Squeeze* 2 sets, 12 reps; whole body 20"
9	*Squeeze* 2 sets, 12 reps	whole body 20"	rest	*Squeeze* 2 sets, 15 reps; whole body 20"
10	*Squeeze* 2 sets, 15 reps	whole body 20"	rest	*Squeeze* 2 sets, 15 reps; whole body 20"
11	*Squeeze* 2 sets, 15 reps	whole body 20"	*Squeeze* 2 sets, 15 reps	*Squeeze* 2 sets, 15 reps; whole body 20"
12	*Squeeze* 2 sets, 15 reps	whole body 20"	*Squeeze* 2 sets, 15 reps	*Squeeze* 2 sets, 15 reps; whole body 20"

Routine B

Week	*Day 1*	*Day 2*	*Day 3*	*Day 4*
1	whole body 15"	*Squeeze* 1 set, 10 reps	rest	*Squeeze* 1 set, 10 reps; whole body 15"
2	whole body 15"	*Squeeze* 1 set, 10 reps	rest	*Squeeze* 1 set, 10 reps; whole body 15"
3	whole body 15"	*Squeeze* 1 set, 10 reps	rest	*Squeeze* 1 set, 10 reps; whole body 18"
4	whole body 18"	*Squeeze* 1 set, 15 reps	*Squeeze* 1 set, 10 reps	*Squeeze* 1 set, 15 reps; whole body 18"
5	*Squeeze* 2 sets, 10 reps	whole body 18"	*Squeeze* 1 set, 10 reps	*Squeeze* 2 sets, 10 reps; whole body 18"

6	*Squeeze* 2 sets, 10 reps	whole body 20"	*Squeeze* 2 sets, 10 reps	*Squeeze* 2 sets, 10 reps; whole body 20"
7	*Squeeze* 2 sets, 12 reps	whole body 20"	*Squeeze* 2 sets, 10 reps	*Squeeze* 2 sets, 12 reps; whole body 20"
8	*Squeeze* 2 sets, 12 reps	whole body 20"; *Squeeze* 2 sets, 12 reps	rest	*Squeeze* 2 sets, 12 reps; whole body 20"
9	*Squeeze* 2 sets, 12 reps	whole body 22"; *Squeeze* 2 sets, 1 rep	rest	*Squeeze* 2 sets 12 reps; whole body 22"
10	*Squeeze* 2 sets, 12 reps	whole body 22"; *Squeeze* 2 sets, 12 reps	rest	*Squeeze* 2 sets, 12 reps; whole body 22"
11	*Squeeze* 2 sets, 12 reps	whole body 22"	*Squeeze* 2 sets, 12 reps	*Squeeze* 2 sets, 12 reps; whole body 25"
12	*Squeeze* 2 sets, 12 reps	whole body 25"	*Squeeze* 2 sets, 12 reps	*Squeeze* 2 sets, 12 reps; whole body 25"

Routine C

Week	*Day 1*	*Day 2*	*Day 3*	*Day 4*
1	whole body 25"; *Squeeze* 1 set, 12 reps	*Squeeze* 1 set, 12 reps	rest	*Squeeze* 1 set, 12 reps; whole body 25"
2	whole body 25"; *Squeeze* 1 set, 12 reps	*Squeeze* 1 set, 12 reps	rest	*Squeeze* 1 set, 12 reps; whole body 25"
3	whole body 25"; *Squeeze* 1 set, 12 reps	*Squeeze* 1 set, 12 reps	rest	*Squeeze* 1 set, 12 reps; whole body 30"

4	whole body 30"	*Squeeze* 1 set, 12 reps	*Squeeze* 1 set, 12 reps	*Squeeze* 1 set, 12 reps; whole body 30"
5	*Squeeze* 2 sets, 10 reps	whole body 30"	*Squeeze* 2 sets, 10 reps	*Squeeze* 2 sets, 10 reps; whole body 30"
6	*Squeeze* 2 sets, 10 reps	whole body 30"	*Squeeze* 2 sets, 10 reps	*Squeeze* 2 sets, 10 reps; whole body 30"
7	*Squeeze* 2 sets, 12 reps	whole body 30"	*Squeeze* 2 sets, 12 reps	*Squeeze* 2 sets, 12 reps; whole body 30"
8	*Squeeze* 2 sets, 12 reps	whole body 35"; *Squeeze* 2 sets, 12 reps	rest	*Squeeze* 2 sets, 12 reps; whole body 35"
9	*Squeeze* 2 sets, 12 reps	whole body 35"; *Squeeze* 2 sets, 12 reps	rest	*Squeeze* 2 sets, 12 reps; whole body 35"
10	*Squeeze* 2 sets, 12 reps	whole body 40"; *Squeeze* 2 sets, 12 reps	rest	*Squeeze* 2 sets, 12 reps; whole body 40"
11	*Squeeze* 2 sets, 12 reps	whole body 40"	*Squeeze* 2 sets, 12 reps	*Squeeze* 2 sets, 12 reps; whole body 40"
12	*Squeeze* 2 sets, 12 reps	whole body 40"	*Squeeze* 2 sets, 12 reps	*Squeeze* 2 sets, 12 reps; whole body 40"

General Pointers

You may use rubber bands or tubing instead of weights, but follow a video from a qualified instructor or learn the proper technique from a fitness professional at your local health club.

If any of the exercises shown feel uncomfortable, feel free to substitute them with others that work the same muscle groups. Remember, this routine should reflect your personal needs and preferences, so feel free to modify it accordingly.

Your Personalised Squeeze Routine

CHART 5: SQUEEZE EXERCISE REFERENCE GUIDE

Exercise Name	Body Part Worked	Page
Squat	thighs, buttocks	64
Squat Kick***	buttocks, thighs	66
Hamstring Curl	thigh	69
Leg Reach	inner thighs, buttocks	70
Calf Raise	calves	71
Inner Thigh Tightener***	inner thigh, buttocks, front and back thighs	72
Gluteal Twist	buttocks and inner thighs	74
Shoulder Raise	shoulders, back	78
Biceps Curl	upper arm, forearms	80
Triceps Press	upper arm	82
Wrist Curl	forearm	84
Rotator Cuff	muscles around the shoulder joint	85
Upper Arm Sculptor***	upper arms	86
Shoulder Row	shoulders, back, upper arms	88
One Arm Row	shoulders, upper and middle back	90
Posture Press	back, shoulders	91
Lower Back Lift	lower back, buttocks	92
Overhead Reach***	back	94
Pullover***	chest and back	95
Seated Row	shoulders and back	96
Back Strengthener***	shoulders, back, buttocks	98
Chest Press	chest, shoulders, upper arm	100
Chest Squeeze	chest, shoulders	102
Posture Push-Up***	chest, upper arms	104
Crunch	abdominals	106
Waist Twist	abdominals	107
Reverse Curl	abdominals	108
Side Lift***	abdominals	109
Reverse Twist***	abdominals	110
Knee Drop***	abdominals	112

***Advanced Exercise

Training Tips

Rest: Realise that rest is a crucial part of your exercise programme. You shouldn't exercise seven days a week, especially if you're just starting out. If you've been working your muscles hard, they need time off to rebuild and become stronger. So relax, take time off and return to each exercise session with lots of energy.

Cross Train: Most fitness injuries are the result of repetitive stress to the same part of the body. If you constantly vary what you do, you'll give your body a break. You may also see quicker improvements in your physique. Once you get used to an activity, your body learns to become more efficient, it learns how to save calories and you have to work a little harder or longer just to keep it challenged. Don't be afraid to try new activities. The fitter you become, the easier they will be for you.

Keep Your Body Guessing: The principle behind exercise is that you challenge your body and it adapts. Once it has adapted you need to challenge it again to see further improvements. Not only can you vary what you do, but you can vary how you do it. If you walk regularly, some days you can walk slowly over a long distance, while other days you may want to alternate walking and jogging. Still other days you may want to focus on walking a mile as fast as possible. Or you can utilise the environment to get you working harder: if you see steps, walk up and down them, walk backwards and sideways, walk up hills, and so on.

Different Days, Different Workouts: The amount of sleep you have had, your mood, diet, any stress you're under and even weather conditions can affect your energy levels. Some days you'll feel stronger than others. Adapt your routine accordingly. If you've had a hard day at work, try a long stretching session instead of your normal routine, for example.

If it's hot you need to acclimatise yourself slowly to the heat and drink plenty of water. Some people worry that drinking water while exercising will cause cramps or nausea. But you can get dehydrated and sick from not drinking water, especially when it is very hot or humid. You should take sips of water at regular intervals before, during and after the exercise period. In cold weather you want to preserve your body heat. Keep your head, hands and feet covered. Since your body may take longer to warm up, move into the activity more slowly than usual.

Pregnancy, medical conditions such as heart ailments or hypertension and some medications may generate an abnormal response to exercise. If these apply to you, seek medical advice first.

Fuel Your Energy Supplies: Exercise will be much harder if you're not getting enough nutrients or calories, your body may not function efficiently and you'll feel tired and listless. Eat plenty of fruit, vegetables and carbohydrates to fuel your energy levels.

Start Slow: If you look for unrealistically quick results, you may do too much too soon, get injured and give up. It's easy to become obsessed for a short while and exercise every day for a couple of weeks. But you'll find your workouts easier and more enjoyable if you start slowly and progress gradually.

Warm up by walking slowly or marching for 5–10 minutes and doing some light stretches. Then, instead of stopping your workout suddenly, slow down gradually to get your heart rate back to normal.

Wait until you're comfortable with your current workload before adding more days or longer exercise periods.

Your Personalised Squeeze Routine

Learn the Basics: If you're uncoordinated in fitness classes or when playing sports, chances are you've just not learned the basic steps properly. If you don't have a health club, sports centre or professional instructor nearby, find books or videos presented by qualified experts. If you have started an activity like tennis or martial arts and realised that your skill level needs to be fairly developed before you can enjoy it, switch modes of exercise. Try something that you can do without having to learn a lot of intricate movements first, like cycling or hiking.

Quality over Quantity: You don't need to spend hours lifting weights to see a difference, it's the *intensity* you work at that matters. If you just want to maintain your current state, you can even decrease your workload a little. As long as you continue at the same exercise intensity during your workouts, you can work out less and not as long. Studies have shown that only when the intensity at which you work out is reduced will you have a measurable decline in your fitness level.

Stay Motivated: The only thing that will guarantee results from an exercise programme is sticking to it. Most people simply do it for a few weeks or months, then give up.

The most important part of your exercise programme is to keep yourself stimulated mentally. You can be motivated by many things: the pressure to win, or to look a certain way, compliments, or the desire to emulate someone you admire. These external sources of motivation can drive you.

To stay inspired, look inside. Address your goals, your needs and your wants. Remind yourself what feels good about exercise and how it helps you. The nice thing about developing this inner motivation is that it takes the effort out of keeping up the exercise habit. If you can change your mind so that you *want* to do it, you won't have to force yourself to. It won't be such a stressful thing trying to remember to do it.

If you miss a few days, don't waste time feeling guilty, get back into your programme and start working out again. Feeling bad about it won't produce results, getting on with it will.

Chapter 13

Losing Fat

Losing Fat

Fat is simply stored energy. Our body breaks it down metabolically so that we can eat, breathe, run, laugh and play. Cellulite is simply another name for fat in the lower body. Although many quack health books and products may try to convince us that cellulite is a serious affliction suffered by women, it's not. It's just fat. It's not a toxic substance, poisoning our bodies, it's just an energy reserve. The only thing wrong with it is our perception. In a different age (circa 1500), you might even be grateful you had the plump, voluptuous look it gives!

What is true is that women tend to have more fat in the lower body, it tends to be closer to the skin (hence it's more visible and more dimply), and it's very hard to lose. Studies have shown that fat in the hips and thighs for women is there for a biological purpose. If you had children during times of famine, you'd be able to call upon all that stored energy for breastfeeding and for the stamina to take care of your young. That said, not many people seem to appreciate it, so they try every method to whittle it away.

You can decrease your body fat significantly, but it does take work. And it does take the right kind and amount of exercise and diet. It's virtually impossible to reshape your body without doing a combination of exercise to both burn calories and build muscle. If you're trying to lose fat, studies have shown that those who do resistance training and aerobic exercise together can lose almost 30 percent more fat than those who do endurance training alone. So the weights you may have been afraid of before suddenly don't look so bad, do they?

Fat is used up by burning calories. Whole body exercises such as aerobics, running, swimming and so on burn the most calories. But whatever you do, you can burn more calories per session just by pushing yourself a little harder – for example, a brisk walk as opposed to an easy walk. By spending more *quality* exercise time, you can often reduce the *quantity* of time but get the same benefits. For example, running 30 minutes burns about the same number of calories as walking for one hour. But working at a harder intensity means you have to be fit to do so. You should not run if you have not built up a good base level of fitness first.

Research has shown that strengthening your muscles is as important as regular aerobic exercise. Not only will you increase the stability of your joints, but you can also thwart the loss of muscle that comes with age. You can develop muscle tone and strength by doing individual exercises such as *The Squeeze* exercises. What most people don't realise is that you will also burn calories while lifting weights. But even more importantly, you will increase your muscle mass. This will help you look firmer and may also increase your metabolism. Finely tuned muscles will give you superb posture, help you move with more grace and precision and help you burn more calories.

The following are some questions I am commonly asked by students and readers.

Which Exercise Burns the Most Calories?

The more muscles you use (arms and legs) and the harder you work determines the amount of calories you burn. If you are carrying your body weight through space it takes even more energy (for example, running vs riding a bike where the bike does some of the work for you). High calorie-burning activities include running, skating, step aerobics, aerobics and cross-country skiing. You can burn more calories during other aerobic activities such as walking, cycling or swimming, if you push yourself a little harder.

Can I Burn Fat From my Thighs, but not my Bum?

Unfortunately we are unable to tell our body where to draw its fat from for energy usage. Generally, fat calories are used from all over the body, but lower body fat in women does seem more resistant. Physiologists speculate that it's because lower body fat is a biological necessity for childbearing.

Can I Burn Calories Without Exercising?

Yes, in fact, calories are simply stored energy in the body. So you always burn calories, whether you are talking, running, or sleeping. All the body's metabolic processes, from cell division to digestion to thinking, require calories to fuel the activity. When you eat you are building up your energy supply by providing more calories to your body.

The problem many women experience is a lowered metabolism after years of dieting. This is known as the 'yo-yo diet syndrome'. The more muscle mass you lose, the fewer calories you burn, so you gain weight much easier. For this reason, it's crucial to exercise if you are dieting and to avoid very low calorie diets. Eat at least 1,200 calories per day.

Why Do I Gain Weight so Easily?

Modern, pre-packaged, high fat foods tend to have many more calories than natural, unprocessed foods. Conveniences like cars and vacuum cleaners mean we don't spend as much time exercising in our daily life any more. Coupled together, the 20th-century person eats more and uses fewer calories than their ancestors. Any calories we don't use get stored as fat for future use. Even if you think you control your food intake, you may be the victim of hidden fats in restaurant and processed foods. Eating fresh foods and being more active *consistently* will help control your weight.

Which Exercise is the Most Fat-burning?

This depends on many things. Generally, you burn more fat by doing high-intensity exercise.

Many people misunderstand fat metabolism. When you exercise, you burn both fat and carbohydrate calories for energy. The ratio of fat and carbohydrates used varies, depending upon many things, including how fit you are, the type of exercise you do, how long you do it for, and so on.

Losing Fat

The fitter you are, the easier it is to burn fat. The less fit you are, the greater your tendency to burn carbohydrates. Since carbohydrate energy stores can run out quickly, you may tire easily when you first begin a fitness programme. Fat is a more efficient fuel source: there's more of it. As you become stronger and fitter your body learns to metabolise fat better so that you can exercise harder and longer.

The confusion arises because how hard you work out can alter your body's choice of fuel. If you exercise fast and hard, you tend to use a higher percentage of carbohydrates (unless you are extremely fit, then your body is able to work harder much more easily and may favour fat). Exercising at a low to moderate intensity means you don't push your body too hard and therefore it isn't forced to use up its quick energy carbohydrates.

But ultimately, for weight loss what is important is *not* the type of calories you burn, but how many overall are used. For example, you can walk for 30 minutes using, say, 200 calories. Since you're not pushing yourself too hard, you may be using a very high percentage of fat. But if you ran hard for 30 minutes and used, say, 300 calories, even though you would have used a lower percentage of fat, your total amount of fat and total overall calories used would be higher.

If you're trying to lose fat, it doesn't really matter where those calories you use come from, for they *both* contribute to weight loss providing you use more than you eat. The general rule is to work as hard as you can in the given amount of time you have to exercise. (But make sure you are working at an intensity that suits your fitness level so that you won't get injured by doing too much too soon. Also, if you are a beginner, you're more likely to stick to exercise if you don't work too hard, so keep that in mind. Six months of consistent exercise is going to do more for you than a couple of very hard workouts.)

If I Diet Do I Still Have to Exercise?

Studies have shown that weight lost from dieting alone is more likely to be regained than if you combine dieting and regular exercise. If you exercise, your dieting will be easier and you don't need to go on a dangerous low calorie diet because you will be using extra calories by working out. The American College of Sports Medicine recommends that you eat at least 1,200 calories a day to meet your daily nutritional and energy needs.

Is Running Dangerous?

Any activity can be dangerous if performed incorrectly. In many respects running is quite safe because the foot hits the ground in the pattern in which it is designed to land: heel to toe. There are also no sudden twists, turns or unnatural joint angles to which the body is subjected. Saying that, running is a very high impact activity so your body must adapt gradually to excessive pounding in order to cope.

Running is one of the highest calorie burners, but you must start gradually and build up your ability to handle the high intensity. Limit the time and frequency of your runs. Start at ten minutes and avoid going longer than 60. Start running two days a week and do no more than five for the safest results. Wear new running shoes and run on soft ground instead of pavement where possible.

It Seems That Now That I'm in my Mid 30s, I Gain Weight More Easily. Why?

Maturity may come with age, but strength doesn't. As you age you can lose 5–6 lb (2.5 kg) of muscle per decade. Because muscle cells require energy, the more you have, the more energy your body requires. Hence, if you have more muscle mass you tend to have a higher metabolism. But *losing* muscle mass means your metabolism slows down too. The result? It's much easier to gain unwanted weight.

Exercise can help thwart the loss of muscle mass that occurs with dieting and ageing, but it's the type of exercise that is key. Studies have shown that aerobic exercise such as walking, stair climbing or cycling can help increase your metabolism temporarily, but won't build lean body tissue (muscle mass). The only type of exercise that actively increases muscle mass is resistance training. Diet with resistance. The answer? Start a resistance-training programme with bands, dumbbells or weight machines *now*.

I've Been Doing Callanetics for Many Months and Have not Lost the Weight From my Thighs. Why?

This is because the small isometric movements used in these 'pulsing' exercises don't burn many calories and don't work a muscle through its full range of motion. Also, it's a myth to think you can spot reduce. Exercise will help reduce fat from your body, but you have no say in where that fat comes from.

I've Heard That High Impact Aerobics can Help You Lose Weight, but That It's Also Dangerous for your Joints. Is This Really True?

High impact aerobics is an excellent calorie-burner, but you must have a good level of fitness before jumping in. The moves do have a lot of impact, but it doesn't have to be stressful. Your foot lands toe to heel during aerobics (rather than heel to toe as when running), so vary your landing moves to avoid repetitive stress on the weaker part, the ball, of your foot. High impact aerobics consists of standard jumping moves like star jumps,

jogging in place, kicks, and so on. So instead of jogging in place for five minutes, then kicking for five minutes, then doing jumping jacks for five minutes, create combinations where you alternate kicks, jogs, and so on every 10–20 seconds. You may also intersperse low impact moves like marching, as opposed to jogging in place, to decrease the pounding force. Like any impact activity, perform it no more than four to five days a week.

Why will I Ultimately Gain Weight From Going on a Very Low Calorie Diet?

When you go on a very low calorie diet (under approximately 1,000–1,200 calories per day), about 25 percent of the weight loss is muscle. The less muscle you have, the fewer calories your body burns during the day. Result? A slower metabolism and easier weight gain. Since most dieters gain all or most of the weight back, when they gain it back they gain it as fat. So the cycle starts: more fat, less muscle, even more fat, even less muscle, and so on. If you lose just 5 lb (2 kg) of muscle you have to eat about 200 fewer calories than you did before to stay at the same weight. The moral? Avoid very low calorie diets and read on.

Can You Burn Calories Lifting Weights?

Yes. Many people are under the false impression that to burn calories you must do vigorous aerobic exercise. In fact, an average weight-lifting workout working all the major muscles in the body can burn about 400 calories an hour. That's the same as walking for the same amount of time. If you do a faster pace circuit workout (where you work your muscles at a fairly high intensity with little rest in between exercises and aerobic-type intervals), you can burn up to 600 calories per hour.

Losing Fat

Can I Really Reshape my Body?

All the marketing hoopla about reshaping your body, thinning your thighs or flattening your abdomen often understates the role of genetics. Simply put, you are born with a predetermined distribution of fat cells and muscle fibre type. But you can enhance what you have by improving your body composition, or muscle to fat ratio. Body reshaping requires that you decrease fat and increase muscle to get physically pleasing proportions. To burn the fat you need to do aerobic exercise such as walking, aerobics or cycling and decrease the fats in your diet. (Strength training will also help burn the calories.) To increase the muscle, what you eat and aerobic activities won't make a difference – you must do resistance training.

Can Stretching Help Me Lose Fat?

Stretching makes you more flexible but it burns about as many calories as sleeping! It can help release tension and improve posture, but cannot by itself decrease your fat stores.

How can I Make my Body Look More Defined?

Muscle definition depends on your muscle mass and body fat levels. Muscles will give you shape. The leaner you are, the more sculpted or 'cut' your muscles will appear because less fat is filling out the curves in your body. Combining calorie-burning exercise with your weight training will help you look more defined by losing fat so you can see the muscles.

Chapter 14

Good Pain, Bad Pain

Good Pain, Bad Pain

An inevitable part of working out is feeling parts of your body you never knew existed. There's just no getting around it; some exercise *does* hurt. But it's important to distinguish between a tired body, an injured muscle, a sore muscle and a painful joint.

Muscle Burning

A burning sensation in your muscles is a sign of depleting energy stores and waste build-up. Providing it stops when you stop the exercise, it is normal and will occur, along with muscular fatigue, towards the end of each set of repetitions. The fitter you are, the longer you can work out without tiring the muscles. If you are doing exercises which target specific muscles, such as sit-ups, leg lifts or arm exercises with weights, the muscle burning is an indication that you have reached a point of fatigue. Relax your muscles, then continue if necessary.

General Fatigue

Overall weakness is a sign that you are tired, dehydrated or depleting your carbohydrate energy stores. You could also be overstressed or overexercising. Rest, because you are more prone to injuries when fatigued. Eat well and drink water before, during and after your workout.

Pain

Since the aim of endurance activities (walking, swimming, aerobics, etc.) is to work all the muscles at once without fatiguing any one group, one muscle getting tired when you are doing a whole body exercise is a sign that you're overdoing it. So if you feel a muscle burning, work out at a lower intensity. If you feel a specific site of pain in a joint, stop exercising immediately, because pain in a specific area, or even a dull ache, can turn into a serious injury. Treat sudden injuries like a twisted ankle or knee right away.

Soreness

You are bound to feel a little bit of soreness in your muscles a day or two after strenuous exercise or when performing a new type of movement. But if you are so sore you have difficulty doing *anything* the next day, you did too much too soon. Decrease the intensity of your next few workouts. If your legs get sore, switch to an upper body workout for a few days, or vice versa. You probably are not allowing enough recovery time in between workouts if you are *continually* sore.

You can minimise the after-effects of a workout by controlling your exercise intensity. For weight loss and fitness benefits you want to work out hard enough to feel challenged, but not uncomfortable. For resistance exercises you want to make sure the muscle you are working feels fatigued at the end of each set, but you don't want to have to huff and puff and strain in order to complete an exercise.

Check Your Technique

Also, make sure that your exercise technique is perfect. Although exercise today is safer than it has ever been, widespread media coverage exaggerating the dangerous elements has given some activities a very bad name (running, aerobics and step, for example). Others are hailed as more gentle, therefore more safe (swimming or yoga). The fact is you can't generalise. *Any* activity can be stressful or safe; it depends upon your technique and your personal fitness level. If you do step aerobics on a step that is too high, you could strain your knees. If you do yoga exercises which strain your already weak back, you could make it worse. If you run before you are fit enough to do so, you may put excess stress on your feet, ankles and knees. Indeed, if you do too much of any exercise before you are ready for it, no matter what it is, you could suffer an injury.

Gyms and fitness classes are carefully designed exercise regimens in a controlled environment. So they would be a safer option for a beginner, providing you are taught by qualified gym and fitness instructors. Activities like sports or dance may be more stressful because all the risky variables like slippery ground, fast-flying objects and unexpected twists can't be controlled.

Exercise to Avoid

Technological advances in exercise science have shown the effects of different movements on the body. And there are certain exercises that most fitness experts recommend the average exerciser not to do.

The rule of thumb is that if an exercise puts potentially harmful stress on a body part, the risks outweigh the benefit of the move. The exercises included in this list are some of the most common exercises in sports and dance training. Full sit-ups, touching your toes while standing, squatting very low on your haunches, double leg lifts while lying on your back, bouncing stretches, the yoga plough, the hurdler stretch and excessive unsupported bending of the spine in any direction are all considered risky.

The problem is most dance classes, yoga routines and sports training warm ups include these moves. Most of them have been practised for centuries. But new research has shown that they can put the body in an *unnecessarily* stressful position. So, while a professional athlete or dancer may have to do some of these moves, experts recommend that most exercisers avoid them. While these movements usually won't cause immediate injuries, they can contribute to wear and tear on the body. Over the long term you could develop a chronic joint problem. Just because you *can* do them, doesn't mean you should.

When in Doubt...

Usually, there are safer alternatives that accomplish the same thing, so there is no need to put your body under undue stress. Your best bet is to seek advice and check up on it periodically to watch for any new developments. Find out from qualified sources: certified fitness instructors, books and videos which are presented by fitness educators with an academic background in the field and current teaching certifications. Don't be fooled by marketing hype. Look for real experts.

The self-awareness you will gain from following *The Squeeze* technique will make you better equipped to listen to your body. When you tune in, you can monitor what feels right or wrong for you. That way you can change a stressful position before it develops into an overuse injury.

The Squeeze technique is safe and more importantly is not just a series of exercises you mimic. You have learned how your body moves; you can now make it stronger and more shapely.

Chapter 15

Now It's Your Turn

Now It's Your Turn

I've given you the formula to sculpt your body. But the real secret to seeing changes in the way you look is to do the exercises regularly.

I hope you have been inspired by this deeper, more substantive view of exercise. Although, undoubtedly, any type of exercise you do will have some effect on your body, I've always believed that time is precious and motivation to exercise is hard to come by. If it's not going to work or if it's going to take a huge amount of effort, why bother? *The Squeeze* will help you see real results in minimal time.

I hope you've also gained a new-found appreciation of how the body works. The body is a wondrous machine with a dazzling capacity to improve itself.

It doesn't take too much to include a fitness regime in your life, and as busy as you are, you'll feel and look better for doing so. Women, in particular, have feared physical strength for a long time. But your strength will bring you confidence that will carry over into other areas of your life.

Most of all I hope that, by learning how to make your exercises more effective and by better understanding what to do, you will be able to integrate fitness naturally into your life so that it becomes a part of it, not some dreaded obligation or brief obsession. By keeping yourself active for the rest of your life, your body will be healthy and strong. You'll have more energy and all your systems will function better. You'll be able to pursue your passions with more vigour and your strength will keep you young beyond your years.

Bibliography

Blakey, Paul, *The Muscle Book*, Bibliotek Books, Stafford, England, 1992.

Brown, D. R., Wang, Y., Ward, A., Ebbeling, C. B., Fortland, L., Puleo, E., Benson, H., and Rippe, J. M., 'Chronic psychological effects of exercise and exercise plus cognitive strategies', *Medicine & Science in Sports & Exercise* 27 (5): 765–75, 1995.

Butts, N. K., and Price, S., 'Effects of a 12-week weight training program on the body composition of women over 30 years of age', *Journal of Strength and Conditioning Research* 8 (4): 265–9, 1994.

Donnelly, Joseph E., EdD, *Living Anatomy*, Human Kinetics Books, Champaign, Illinois, second edition, 1990.

Ellison, Deborah, PT, 'Functional flexibility', *IDEA Today*, May 1995.

Enoka, Roger M., *Neuromechanical Basis of Kinesiology*, Human Kinetics Publishers, Champaign, Illinois, second edition, 1988.

Harris, Dorothy, PhD, and Harris, Bette L., EdD, *Sports Psychology: Mental Skills for Physical People*, Leisure Press, Champaign, Illinois, 1984.

Hoffman, Stephanie, MS, PT, and Franchis, Lorna, PhD, 'Is balance missing from your workout?', *IDEA Today*, March 1992.

Kapit, Wynn, and Elson, Lawrence M., *The Anatomy Coloring Book*, Harper & Row Publishers, New York, 1977.

Kubistant, Tom, EdD, *Mind Pump: The Psychology of Bodybuilding*, Leisure Press, Champaign, Illinois, 1988.

LaChance, Peter F., and Hortobagyi, Tibor, 'Influence of cadence on muscular performance during push-up and pull-up exercise', *Journal of Strength and Conditioning Research* 8 (2): 76–9, 1994.

La Forge, Ralph, 'Research', *IDEA Today*, September 1992.

La Forge, Ralph, '1995 Research', *IDEA Today*, October 1995.

Luttgens, Kathryn, PhD, and Wells, Katharine F., PhD, *Kinesiology: Scientific Basis of Human Motion*, Saunders College Publishing, New York, seventh edition, 1982.

McComas, A. J., 'Human neuromuscular adaptations that accompany changes in activity', *Medicine & Science in Sports & Exercise* 26 (12): 1498–1509, 1994.

Monroe, Mary, ed., 'Industry News', *IDEA Today for the Fitness Professional*, Nov/Dec 1990.

Monroe, Mary, 'This year in research', *IDEA Today*, October 1994.

Morgan, W. P., 'Psychological components of effort sense', *Medicine & Science in Sports & Exercise* 26 (9): 1071–7, 1994.

Richmond, Phyllis G., MA, 'The Alexander Technique and dance training', *Impulse: The International Journal of Dance Science, Medicine and Education* 2 (1): 24–38, 1994.

Rothenberg, Beth and Oscar, *Touch Training for Strength*, Human Kinetics Publishers, Champaign, Illinois, 1995.

Ruther, C. L., Goldend, C. L., Harris, R. T., and Dudley, G. A., 'Hypertrophy, resistance training, and the nature of skeletal muscle activation', *Journal of Strength and Conditioning Research* 9 (3) 155–9, 1995.

Signorile, J. F., Weber, B., Roll, B., Caruso, J., Lowensteyn, I., and Perry, A. C., 'An electromyographical comparison of the squat and knee extension exercises', *Journal of Strength and Conditioning Research* 8 (3): 178–83, 1994.

Tenenbaum, G., Bar-Eli, M., Hoffman, J. R., Jablonovski, R., Sade, S., and Shitrit, D., 'The effect of cognitive and somatic psyching-up techniques on isokinetic leg strength performance', *Journal of Strength and Conditioning Research* 9 (1): 3–7, 1995.

Weinberg, Robert S., PhD, *The Mental Advantage: Developing Your Psychological Skills in Tennis*, Leisure Press, Champaign, Illinois, 1988.

Westcott, Wayne, PhD, *Strength Fitness: Physiological Principles and Training Techniques*, fourth edition, WCB Brown & Benchmark Publishers, Madison, Wisconsin, 1995.

Wilmore, Jack H., PhD, and Costill, David L., PhD, *Physiology of Sport and Exercise*, Human Kinetics Publishers, Champaign, Illinois, 1994.

Recommended Reading

Bean, Anita, *Sports Nutrition*, The Crowood Press, 1993.

Heaner, Martica, *CURVES – The Body Transformation Strategy*, Hodder & Stoughton, 1995.

Heaner, Martica, *The 7 Minute SEX Secret*, Coronet, 1995.

Kubistant, Tom, EdD, *Mind Pump: The Psychology of Bodybuilding*, Leisure Press, 1988.

Langer, Ellen J., PhD, *Mindfulness*, Harvill.

Newby-Fraser, Paula, with Mora, John M., *Peak Fitness for Women*, Human Kinetics, 1995.

Smith, Bob, *Flexibility for Sport*, The Crowood Press, 1994.

Vartabedian, Roy, and Matthews, Kathy, *Nutripoints*, Grafton, 1990.

Order Martica's other books and videos!

Books:

CURVES – The Body Transformation Strategy
CURVES shows you *exactly* how to achieve your personal goal: decrease fat, resculpt your physique, increase your energy, improve your health or just relax and experience peace through movement. Learn more about weight loss, injury, fat, muscle, motivation, exercise myths and more! Discover the perfect exercise plan for you, then learn how to stick to it so you see results (available from Hodder & Stoughton, 338 Euston Road, London, NW1 3BH and in leading bookstores near you).

The 7 Minute SEX Secret
All women are advised to do pelvic floor exercises from an early age. What better motivation than an improved sex life? Learn how the muscles work and exercises to develop strength and stamina in the love muscles. Recommended by leading physiotherapists (available From Hodder & Stoughton, 338 Euston Road, London NW1 3BH and in leading bookstores near you).

Secrets of an Aerobics Instructor
If you are interested in becoming a fitness teacher, this book gives you insights into how to develop, analyse and improve your instructing skills and techniques.

How To Be A Personal Trainer
If you are interested in entering the lucrative field of personal fitness training, use this manual to start up. Includes fitness, business and marketing ideas.

Videos:

THE SQUEEZE Arms & Abs Workout
A calming but intense body sculpting workout featuring Martica's mind–body *Squeeze* technique. Focuses on the upper body to improve your posture and help you get firm, flat abs.

THE SQUEEZE Butt & Thighs Workout
A mind–body muscle sculpting workout featuring Martica's *Squeeze* technique. Focuses on the lower body to lift and shape the buttocks and tone the thighs.

Martica's SEXY BODY Workout
An invigorating and stimulating workout to get your whole body ready for great sex! Target the buttocks, hips and thighs. Develop flexibility from easy stretches. Increase your stamina in an energy-increasing aerobics routine. Develop perfect pelvic muscle control and firm up your sex muscles with Sex Squeezes!

Martica's PERFECT CURVES Workout
This video offers you a blend of hi-lo moves and bodysculpting exercises with weights. Burn fat, increase energy levels, strengthen your hips, thighs, buttocks, abdominals and upper body. Easy to follow.

Thighs, Tums and Bums
Burn fat calories by CardioSculpting – low impact aerobics with tough leg work for your hips and thighs. Also includes a flattening abdominal section. Simple moves and clear explanations make this workout good for men and beginners as well as experienced exercisers. Given top reviews by leading magazines and papers.

Order Form

Name _____

Address _____

_____

Postcode: _____   Tel: _____

Please send _____ copies of *The Squeeze Arms & Abs Workout* video @ £12.99 each   £ _____

Please send _____ copies of *The Squeeze Butt & Thighs Workout* video @ £12.99 each   £ _____

Please send _____ copies of *PERFECT CURVES Workout* video @ £12.99 each   £ _____

Please send _____ copies of *Martica's SEXY BODY Workout* video @ £12.99 each   £ _____

Please send _____ copies of *Thighs, Tums and Bums* low impact video @ £12.99 each   £ _____

Please send _____ copies of *Secrets* @ just £16.99 each   £ _____

Please send _____ copies of *Personal Trainer* @ just £14.99 each   £ _____

All prices include p+p in the UK; countries outside the UK add £5.00 per item   £ _____

Credit Cards accepted: VISA/MC/Access/Eurocard/JCB   Total Amount: £ _____

Number _____   Expiry _____

Signature _____

Make cheque/PO payable to Mind & Muscle.
Send order to PO Box 363, Dept HH, London WC2H 9BW

Credit card hotline: 0171 240 9861

Suppliers

Where to Get Weights

You should be able to find light weights at your nearest sports store. I would suggest buying solid dumbbells in individual sizes. There are some which are adjustable, allowing you to add on extra weight. These are often less secure; it's better just to get several pairs of varying sizes. Dumbbells range from £5–£15 a pair, depending on the size. I would recommend starting off with two or three pairs so that you can switch the amount of weight you use depending upon the exercise. Try a 1 lb or 2 lb (0.5 kg or 1 kg) pair and a 3 lb or 4 lb (1.5 kg or 2 kg) pair.

Weider Weights are an excellent brand. You can obtain them from the following retail outlet or through mail order:

Physical Company
Cherry Cottage
Hedsor Road
Bourne End
Buckinghamshire
SL8 5DH

Tel: 01628 520208

Other Fitness Products

The Step and Body Bar
Forza Fitness Equipment
Fourth Floor
Europe House
The World Trade Centre
London
E1 9AA

Tel: 0171 488 9488

The Fitness Pro-Mat
Beacons Products Ltd
Fitness Pro-Mat m/b
Unit 10
EFI Industrial Estate
Brecon Road
Merthyr Tydfil
CF47 8RB

Tel: 01685 350 011